NATURAL FLOW

A Woman's Guide to Menstrual Health

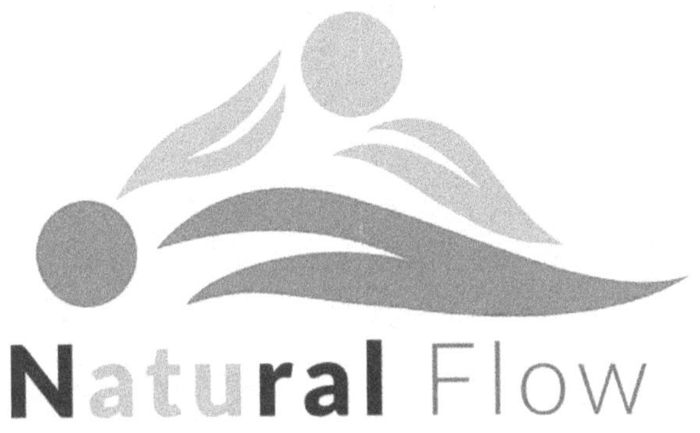

By Dr. Dean Fitzgerald

Natural Flow:

- Free One-On-One Consultation
  Spend 20-30 minutes to discuss how we
  can help you
- Everyone who applies for a consultation
  receives a gift

4 WAYS TO REGISTER

Mobile Text
Text to: 58885 your name and email with the
keyword "**Flow**"

Voice
Call 866-603-3995 PIN # 149400

Web
www.bonus.Naturalflowforwomen.com

QR Code

Table of Contents

Dedication

This book is dedicated to…

My amazing, beautiful wife Doris. She has stood beside me and put up with all my craziness for the last 35 years. Without her I am very certain my life would be in a much different place right now.

ACKNOWLEDGEMENT…

For several years I've had this idea bouncing around in the back of my head to write a book and open a specialty clinic to help women. I was always so tied up with what I was already doing, and, quite honestly, wasn't sure where to start, that it just never happened! Then one day I was at a totally unrelated conference and met Cevin and Mark. Cevin is a best-selling author, and Mark works in the marketing industry. Their example finally flipped the "get it done" switch in my head. Thank you Cevin and Mark.

I also must thank Barry Schimmel who has patiently given me the step-by-step methods to complete this work. Having the information in my head, and actually putting that information into an organized, usable format are two entirely different accomplishments. Barry's guidance has allowed me to mesh the two. Thank you Barry.

Finally, and most importantly, I must thank my beautiful wife Doris, our 6 Daughters, and our 17 grandchildren for giving me the inspiration to do what I do. It is for them that I try to improve the world in which we live.

Dr. Dean Fitzgerald

Dean's Story

Dean Fitzgerald started his working career in the oilfields of eastern Utah. Being somewhat taken back by the unpredictability of that work environment, he decided a little later in life to change careers. He eventually graduated from Palmer College of Chiropractic, Davenport IA and started a solo practice in the fall of 1998.

During the past 19 years of practice Dr. Fitzgerald has helped thousands of patients, and administered 10's of thousands of treatments.

Dr. Fitzgerald graduated in the top of his class. -He has been nominated many times for the Who's Who of healthcare -He spent 9 ½ years in the air national guard. -He worked for 7 years on his home town's city council. -Together with his wife raised 6 daughters.

Message to the World

I am the solution you've been looking for to normalize your menstrual cycles; reduce painful cramping; normalize flow; regulate cycles; help with hormonal regulation; help with getting pregnant; help with headaches and with low back pain. Normal pain free cycles lead to a much happier life.

Message intended for:

Women of all ages that are experiencing irregular or painful menstrual cycles or are trying to get pregnant.

Two things about me:

1) I get to the cause of the problem. I don't just cover it up with medications, or cut it out. Essentially, I fix the problem, so the body can normalize itself.
2) I specialize in women's health and do it all naturally with amazing results.

Give back attitude:

I consistently continue my education to learn more and improved techniques which increases my overall success.

Purpose

My purpose is to improve the lives of as many people as possible - not just today, but for generations to come as well.

Chapter 1: **Symptoms**

Your symptoms can be stopped

Painful Menstrual Cycles

It is absolutely mind boggling the number of women that dread their cycles every month because of pain. These women complain of everything from cramping and bloating to nausea and headaches. Some women say that suddenly their legs weigh a thousand pounds each. Some state that they are so sick every month that they don't eat for days. Some ladies don't even realize that all the pain they are experiencing is directly related to the hormonal changes that occur within their own bodies every month. These painful symptoms can be stopped, and this book's goal is to explain how. In the next few sections let's examine some of the symptoms a little more closely.

Painful Tailbone (Coccyx)

Have you ever fallen hard into a seated position? Have you ever wrecked a bicycle in a way that caused you to slip forward and straddle the bar in front of the seat? Have you ever landed on the edge of the trampoline by accident? Has anyone of your friends ever playfully kicked you a little too hard in the bottom? If any of these things, or a hundred other similar things, has happened to you, it is likely you have experienced some sort of pain in the tailbone (or Coccyx) region. Unfortunately, many of types of injuries occur and are never properly treated. Later I will discuss how these injuries can, and do, affect natural menstrual cycles. Just know for now that present, or history of, pain in the tailbone (Coccyx) can, and many times does, lead to abnormal menstruation.

Irregular Menstrual Cycles

What is 'irregular'? I guess to answer that question one needs to know what 'regular' is. So, let's define regular then realize that anything other than regular is irregular. An average regular menstrual cycle in healthy women occurs every 28 days – thus the word cycle. For the purposes of this discussion I will break the 28-day cycle into two-time frames – days 1-14 and days 15-28. I should point out again that 28 days is an average among women, and can vary depending on what is occurring in any given woman's life at the time. However, the general phases should remain about the same with the exception being in the duration.

The menstrual cycle is commonly counted as starting on the first day of menstruation. This is the beginning of two simultaneous events. The first is the sluffing off the fluid engorged lining of the uterus. The only place for this fluid and lining tissue to exit is through the vaginal opening. Women commonly state that they have started their periods when this begins. Sluffing of the uterine wall generally last about 5 days with menstruation lasting about 7 days as the last of the menstrual fluid is finally expelled. Women often state that they have just finished their period when fluid flow stops. During this 7-day period the uterine muscles and the abdominal muscles will contract to help expel the uterine wall and associated fluids. This contraction should be just that – a contraction! The contraction is noticeable, but not major, long lasting cramps that make the woman want to shut down life for the next 7 days.

Now, I said two events were occurring during the first 14 days. The second of these events is the development of a mature egg within the ovary. Hormones are released which trigger the ovary to begin the egg development process. This takes 14 days with the egg being released on the fourteenth day. After being released, the egg is pulled into the fallopian tube. This process is called ovulation. Some women state that they feel a slight sharp or tearing pain when the egg is released. Some ladies even state that they will feel a little sensation of achiness for a short time afterwards. These sensations are normal, but should be just that – sensations.

Also occurring during the second half of the first 14 days is the healing and rebuilding of the uterine wall lining.

Ovulation marks the beginning of the second half of the menstrual cycle. Once in the fallopian tube the mature egg only last about 24 hours while it waits to meet up with a sperm cell to start pregnancy. The hormones in the body keep the uterine wall engorged and ready to receive a fertilized egg to begin the process of growing a baby. If this does not happen, the hormones once again change and triggers the stopping of the engorgement of the uterine wall. This leads to the uterine wall breaking down and the process begins all over again.

During this second half of the menstrual cycle it is common for women to retain a little extra fluid throughout their bodies. This is normal as the body prepares to lose fluid during menstruation. This fluid retention may present as a slight bloated feeling or a slight swollen feeling. The feelings of bloat and swelling should not dominate one's life just prior to the beginning of their period.

Now, with all that said, the thing to get from this discussion is the fact that any deviation from the described cycle is "irregular"! I will discuss a few of these deviations, or irregularities, in the next few sections.

Excessive Flow

In the previous section I alluded to the hormones changing at various times during the 28-day cycle. If these hormones change to the excess, then the result will be an excess of whatever that hormone was meant to trigger. At this point I could go into a lengthy discussion of which hormones do what as the menstrual cycle progresses, but that is not what is important here. What the reader should understand is that her menstrual cycle is, for the most part, dictated by hormone levels in her body. Too much or too little hormones at certain times during the cycle will negatively affect the menstrual cycle. Excessive flow is often caused by too much hormones at certain times and too little hormones at other times.

No Flow

No flow is caused by more factors then excessive flow. No flow can be caused by hormones, or it can be caused by life style changes. Some high performing athletes notice a huge reduction, or complete cessation, of menstrual flow. Increased stress or trauma can cause no flow. What the reader should understand is that most commonly no flow is also related to hormone production or the lack there of.

Wi-Fi

At this point the reader should be asking, "How do I control my hormone production?" which is a very good question. The easiest way for me to explain this is by comparing the hormones of the body to a Wi-Fi signal. Wi-Fi is generally broadcast to a certain area such as a business or home. Many people go to their favorite coffee shop to connect and get something done while sipping their morning wakeup.

If we look at the bigger picture, we will see that the Wi-Fi is controlled by the copper or fiber hard lines that service the building or area they are in. Those hard lines transmit all the information to and from the Wi-Fi inside the defined area. The information is channeled to a central hub. That hub is connected to millions of other hubs throughout the world in a system that we call the internet.

A similar system exists within our bodies. You see, the hormones are like the Wi-Fi they are secreted from multiple different glands in the body and circulate to be used by whichever organ needs them. However, the glands are hard wired to a central hub called the brain. The hard wiring is called the nervous system. If the hard wiring to your coffee shop is affected, then the Wi-Fi will be affected. Likewise, if your nervous system is affected then the glands that produce hormones will also be affected. With this understanding, let's move on to some other symptoms that are possible during an irregular menstrual cycle.

Endometriosis

Endometriosis is a term often used to describe an inflammation of the lining of the uterine wall. A more specific word would be endometritis. While endometriosis refers to inflammation within the pelvic cavity, endometritis refers to inflammation of the uterus wall specifically. None-the-less, the inflammation of the uterine wall is the problem. This inflammation can wreak havoc on a woman's life. Great pain and cramping, and whole-body achiness are only a couple of the associated symptoms. What the reader needs to remember here is that endometritis or endometriosis is the symptom not the problem.

Headaches during menstrual cycle

In our world of healthcare, it has become the normal accepted practice to break the body's systems into specialties. For example, there are Cardiologist, Oncologists, Nephrologist, Neurologist, Urologist, Dermatologist, Gynecologist, etc., etc., etc. And although I believe it is very important to specialize, and become expert, in each field, we mustn't lose sight of the bigger picture which is overall health. About now the reader is probably asking themselves, "What does this have to do with headaches?" The answer to that question is quite simple. When a woman experiences menstrual headaches, she is referred to a specialist. This specialist is familiar with menstrual cycle issues, but the problem in his or her eyes is in the head not the reproductive system – thus the term 'headache. Rarely would such a specialist refer the patient to a Gynecologist, and if they do, the Gynecologist doesn't specialize in headaches. Somehow with all our modern technology, we've lost sight of the overall picture. It is amazing how many women suffer from monthly headaches. I will discuss a little later how to solve this problem and how to get women the relief they need from their headaches.

Inability to Get Pregnant

As I write this section there are many reasons that come to mind as to why a woman who would like to start a family is unable to. Because I have discussed hormones, let's start there. What would happen if the hormone that triggered the release of the mature egg was never secreted? What if the hormone that triggered the engorgement of the uterine wall was too low? What if the hormones were secreted in the opposite order?

Remember the hard wiring to the glands? What if the signals from the brain were so impeded on the hard wiring that the Fallopian tubes were unable to get the hormonal and neurological signal to tell them to pull the egg in?

These are just a few of the possible reasons. Please understand that all these things can be corrected in most healthy women. I will discuss these issues in another section later in the book.

Symptoms Summary

One of my goals with this introductory chapter is to get the reader to expand her thinking. So often we explain abnormalities away to normalize them. I'm here to tell you that menstrual health problems and their associated symptoms are NOT normal. But more importantly, there is help if you look in the right place. This book is a good start. In the next chapter, I will discuss some of the common treatments and some of the reasons they often don't work as hoped.

Chapter 2: **Common Treatments**

Medications

The number one first answer to anybody's symptoms, of any kind, in our society today is to send them to their pharmacy. There are medications that medicate the patient against medications! It is nearly un-real the amounts of drugs that are prescribed daily. Now I don't mean to sound like all drugs are bad, but, again, I feel we should look at the bigger picture. One question that should always be asked when a medication is prescribed for a treatment is, "How, exactly, will the medication work?"

We are so symptom based in our world that often getting rid of the symptom comes at the expense of future health.

Let's use the topic at hand – menstrual health (or un-health). Cramping is a common symptom, so I'll chose it. Think about this now! When a patient goes to their Ob-Gyn because of cramping their goal is to stop the cramping -right? About now I envision every reader saying, "duh!" Well, bear with me. Remember I said the cramping was a symptom? The real question should be, "what caused the symptom – cramping?" Is the answer because too much hormones were secreted? Is the answer because the hard wiring to the glands have been impeded? Is the answer because ___________? You could fill in the blank with lots of other reasons. So, in asking the question of how exactly the medication works, we are demanding of the prescribing doctor to voice his or her diagnosis of what the actual problem is.

You see, if the prescribing doctor thinks the problem is in the gland itself, then the medication should be aimed at repairing the gland. Wouldn't you agree? Often this is not the case. Often patients complain of cramping, so the doctor prescribes a medication that will cause the muscles to decrease their contraction in the hopes that the cramping will lesson or stop. I'm telling you that the cramping is often only a symptom of other problems. If the other problems are taken care of then the cramping (the symptom) will quit.

An analogy I like to use involves your car. Let's say you jump into your car with some of the people in your life that are close to you and head for your favorite restaurant. As you pull out of your driveway, you look down and notice that the low oil warning light has come on. There are many situations within the overall function of your car that could cause the light to illuminate. Some of those things could include a leak in the oil pan; the last oil change being short on replacement oil; the car could have started burning oil; the oil pump may be going out and not properly working; the oil level sensor could be broken; etc. Just to name a few. However, the symptom that you are concerned about is the illuminated light.

At this time, you remember that just a block over from the route you are on is a mechanic's shop with a mechanic that you trust. When you tell the mechanic about your light, he or she politely listens then grabs a small can of black paint. With paint in hand the mechanic goes over to your car and removes the clear front portion of your dashboard and proceeds to spray black paint over the illuminated light until it is no longer visible. He or she then replaces the dashboard and hands you a bill for services. Now remember, your concern was the illuminated light! The light is now no longer visible. The mechanic did exactly as you wanted and fixed your symptom.

The question in this scenario is, "Did painting over the light fix the cause of the light illuminating?" Obviously, the answer is no it did not! Unfortunately, the same is often true when it comes to medications – they just cover up the symptom until something more serious occurs. Although the symptom may lesson or be relieved, the medication often does little or nothing to fix the actual cause of the problem.

Hysterectomy

I will start this section by saying that there are a few situations that do warrant a hysterectomy being done. For example, occasionally women will have babies and for various reasons the suspensory ligaments fail, and their uteruses prolapse. If the surgeon doesn't feel that repairing the ligaments is a viable solution, then hysterectomy is the only option. Another instance would be uterine cancer. Obviously, hysterectomy to save a woman's life is a wise choice. Sever trauma, or multiple caesarean sections could also lead to hysterectomy. That said, the majority of surgeries to remove the uterus are performed because the medications didn't work. In other words, the Ob-Gyn has limited options, and when the options are exhausted protocol dictates hysterectomy as his or hers next step. Removing the problem altogether will certainly stop the symptoms, but at what expense?

In the last section, I used the analogy of painting over the oil light. In the case of hysterectomy, instead of covering the light the mechanic just opens the hood and takes the engine out. Again, the symptom of an illuminated oil light is solved. Of course, the car is now missing a vital part that is need for its overall function. I'm here to tell you that keeping your uterus is also needed for your overall function.

In the next chapter, I'll explain some of the lasting complications of hysterectomy. Then later in the book I will introduce a much more viable option.

Tailbone Removal (Coccygectomy)

This surgery is performed because of tailbone pain that is non-relieving. This symptom is a difficult one to treat. Unless the treating physician knows just how to deal with it, the patient may go years with the pain. I can understand why ladies would consent to having the tailbone removed. I often wonder what I would do after months, or even years, of annoying, sometimes unbearable, pain.

But, again, I urge the reader to look at the bigger picture. The tailbone in and of itself is not the problem. Removing the tailbone may reduce the pain, but I must repeat the question - at what expense? Additionally, I would ask what the real cause of the pain is. I will discuss a little later the actual cause and what I can do to help ladies relieve the tailbone pain they are struggling with.

Physical Therapy

I personally believe that a good physical therapist is worth their weight in gold. If the physical therapist understands the human body to the point of actually being able to see the cause and effect of various conditions, then he or she can nearly work miracles. Too often; however, physical therapists use a cookie cutter approach. Too often a patient presents with certain symptoms, and the therapist just refers to the text book treatment like he she learned in school. Thankfully, for a great deal of the

patients, this technique gives some relief. My concern is for the patients that this approach doesn't work. Unfortunately, that percentage is much too great.

In our society healthcare has become somewhat of a funnel. While the top of the funnel is wide, if you fall into it the way out is through the small end which generally represents a surgery. Physical therapists are somewhere about half or three quarters of the way down the funnel. If their treatment doesn't work, then the patient is just pushed a little closer to the small opening at the end of the funnel.

Certainly, most patients don't enter healthcare with a hope to have surgery. And, although that may be the case, when the surgeon says, "it's time to go under the knife" few people look for other options. Well I'm here to tell you that if physical therapy doesn't work for your tailbone pain, or menstrual cramping, etc. there is another treatment, that has high success, available.

Message

If you've read the book up to this point, I must assume that you are one of those People who are looking for an answer to one or more of the symptoms described in the first chapter. I'm also going to step out on a limb and guess that you've tried a treatment or two with limited success. If my assumptions are correct (or not), then the question I have for you is, "have you thought of or tried massage?" Think about it, if you are experiencing severe cramping, or constant pain, etc., then getting the muscles to relax could give you some much needed relief. Who wouldn't want a brief reprieve from the misery? I've known patients that were able to have a few days of less pain and better sleep after a good, blissful massage.

 Although massage is wonderful, it is seldom a cure. That said, the benefits of massage come with essentially no side effects, and the patient can have some longer periods of relief while arranging other treatment plans.

Meditation

Before beginning this book, I did a search on the internet to see what ladies were doing for their menstrual cycle disorders. I was surprised to see the amount of information relating to meditation. Personally, I believe our minds have the power to heal us. I honestly believe that if a person could learn to control their thoughts, and become in tune with their bodies, they could greatly improve their health overall. However, that level of controlled thought is difficult to achieve, and relatively few individuals are able to do so. With this knowledge in mind, I would encourage the reader to spend time daily in quiet meditation. You will find that life's challenges become more manageable if you spend 30 minutes of alone time each day. Now that doesn't mean to take a 30-minute nap. Nor does it mean to spend 30 minutes catching up on phone calls or this week's Facebook posts. This 30 minutes of meditation is to be spent alone quietly discovering the energy within your own body. Some people start by concentrating on their feet and feeling every square inch of each foot in their minds. Then they work their way up to the legs then hips, etc. In part, this exercise improves the brain's communication with the rest of the body. The act of focusing on specific parts of the body and feeling what they are doing is performed by the nervous system. Our nervous systems are similar to the rest of our bodies in that if it is not used it slowly wastes away. Additionally, by improving the communication between our bodies and our brains, our brain can detect any potential health problems earlier and thus begin the healing process earlier.

Another benefit of daily meditation is that subtle thoughts will come to the meditator that will help guide their daily decisions. Listen to these thoughts and study them in your own mind so that you can discover if and how they apply to you. Remember, the goal of meditation is to improve your overall life.

There have been volumes upon volumes of writings about meditation by people much more qualified than me. I would suggest that if you're interested in meditation as a healing source that you seek out a trained professional to guide you along the way.

For the purposes of this book, I would recommend that you read to the end to discover a treatment for menstrual conditions that won't take the years required to do it through meditation. Please remember that meditation is a very productive use of one's time and can be, and should be, done in conjunction with other treatment protocols.

Barely touched the surface

It is next to impossible to stay abreast of all the treatments available for all the various conditions that affect menstrual health. What the reader should understand is that there are too many factors involved in the decision-making process of which treatment to administer. Additionally, outside forces such as professional organizations and insurance companies play a role in a health care provider's recommended treatment. Due to these, and many other, factors, the best treatment for a given illness may never be administered to the patient.

At my clinic, the goal is, and always has been, on the patient. I administer what I feel is the most appropriate treatment to heal the patient. I really don't expend much energy towards satisfying the bureaucracy. I truly wish that all healthcare professionals were able to do the same.

In the next chapter, I will point out some of the long-term effects of the common treatments that that I just discussed.

Chapter 3: How Do You Wish to Live the Rest of Your Life?

Deep Desires

As I read back through my notes for this chapter, I realized that it all seemed like doom and gloom. Obviously, my goal is not to depress the reader, but to spread some hope. I ask you, the reader, to keep in mind that you have choices, and knowing some of the long-term results of these choices can help in the decision-making process.

You see, I earnestly believe that most peoples' deepest desires are to live a long, healthy, and fulfilling life. I believe that most people, ladies especially, wish to be a force for good on this earth. I also know that negative health issues can create a huge barricade in one's life moving towards these worthy desires. Unfortunately, there exists conditions in life that are somewhat bleak, but must be talked about. With that in mind, please read the following sections for informational and decision-making purposes.

Medications

In the previous chapter I used the example of painting over the low oil warning light. I realize that example is not something that mechanics do on a regular basis. But, I have a friend that took his car to a couple of different mechanic shops where they couldn't find the problem as to why the "check engine" light came on. Eventually, the mechanic told him he could unplug the light under the dashboard. – TRUE STORY!

Unfortunately, many health care professionals are like the mechanics mentioned above. They are hardworking; well-meaning doctors that just can't figure out what the actual problem is. In fact, our healthcare delivery system has become mostly a reactionary treatment system.

What I mean by that is, if a patient presents with symptoms A, B, and C, then medication D is prescribed. If medication D doesn't work, then medication E is prescribed. If the second medication doesn't work, then either medication F is prescribed, or the patient is sent to a specialist who in turn prescribes medication F. This becomes a vicious cycle until the symptoms become worse than the medications can cover up. The next step, of course, is to just cut out the symptomatic organ and not have to deal with it any more. Notice that nowhere along the way is the cause of the symptoms addressed! If the patient is astute enough to ask what caused the symptoms, they are told that sometimes these things just happen – lucky you!

Well my question is, "do you want to spend a great deal of, or the rest of, your life stuck in that vicious cycle?" Wouldn't it be much better to solve the cause of the symptom rather than just cover it up? I assure you that it is very unlikely that the cause of the symptoms is a lack of the medication in your body. The symptoms you are experiencing is your body's way of dealing with whatever the cause is. If those symptoms are artificially stopped, or covered up, your body must react in a different way. Often the different way is worse than the symptom that is being covered up in the first place. And, just like the car example, later on the cause of the symptom will be much harder, take more time, and be much more expensive to treat.

I have a neighbor that many years ago came to see me because of debilitating headaches, especially during her menstrual cycle. I examined her and discovered the cause of her headaches. When I explained to her the best treatment to correct the cause of her headaches, she told me that the time required was more than she could do at that point. Additionally, her insurance wouldn't cover all the care, so she went back to the medications (which the insurance paid for).

Since that time, she has had multiple surgeries. One of the surgeries was to implant a device that she could turn on when the headaches were too bad, and the electrical shock would override the pain in her head and reduce the headache. The next surgery was to remove that implanted device when it didn't work as hoped. All along the way her medications have become more potent and the dosage has increased. About 15 years have passed, and during that time she has occasionally visited my clinic. Each time she comes in, I tell her the same thing. And, although she has had good intentions, she still will not commit to the short care program that I feel will help her.

In closing this section, I would ask the reader to look around to their friends and family. How many of these people have been through similar treatments to my neighbor's over the years? Are you looking forward to the same lifestyle? Do you want to finally be overcome by the symptoms and feel there is no other way? I have had many patients over the years with similar symptoms to my neighbor's that are now living healthy, productive, fulfilling lives. There is a good chance That I could help with the cause of your symptoms also.

Hormone Replacement Medications

A healthy woman's uterus and ovaries, along with various glands within the body, produce and regulate the hormones throughout her body. These hormones are released in just the right amounts at just the right time to make her body function properly. This is especially true when it comes to having proper menstrual cycles. Could you imagine trying to constantly monitor all the hormone levels and adding a little here and a little there to keep the whole system functioning at top performance? To consciously perform such a feat with success would literally consume one's entire day each and every day! So how is it that hormone replacement medications can do it? The answer is – They are not able!

Now I know there are thousands—no, tens of thousands of women that have had complete hysterectomies and are doing okay with the replacement hormones they are taking. That said, how dare I make such a statement as to say the replacement hormones don't keep the body functioning? Allow me to elaborate. I will be the first to tell you that if a woman has undergone a complete hysterectomy, then the replacement hormones are a god-send. But, those hormones, at best, keep the levels in the body elevated so that the rest of the hormone producing glands must react to them. Many times, this has caused the other glands to become overstressed. Usually the prescribing doctor monitors the patient with blood work etc. to adjust the hormone replacement medication's dosage to best fit the patient's demands. But, even with this careful monitoring, it is all but impossible to get it perfect.

Think about it! A woman's body can monitor her hormone levels 24 hours a day, 7 days a week. Her body also can add a little bit of natural hormones here and there to keep all the levels within the normal balance.

However, with hormone replacement medications, the same women takes her pills only at given times throughout the day. Therefore, there must be extra medication available when the body needs it. Often this elevated level of hormones causes other hormones to elevate, which, in turn, can cause various other symptoms in the patient. For example, minor bouts of anxiety, depression, anger, hot or cold flashes, etc. Sometimes skin eruptions will appear, or hair will be a little extra oily. Perhaps the patient will experience water retention roller coasters. These symptoms can be credited to the body trying to regulate its hormones. The obvious question at this point is, "do you, the reader, look forward to dealing with a life filled with these ups and downs?" Do you look forward to having to remember to take your pills at the same time every day for the rest of your life? Wouldn't you rather do whatever you can to try and solve the cause of the symptoms rather than just cover them up or cut them out?

At this point I need to tell you about a woman who was a great influence in my life. She has passed away now, but she played a tremendous role in making me the person I am today. One of the greatest roles was in raising my wife. All the clichés about mothers-in-law were one hundred percent wrong when it came to my mother-in-law. She truly was an amazing, loving woman.

When her and my father-in-law were first married, they experienced financial struggles just as many young couples do. These struggles lead to her looking for work to help pay for the family's needs. As the story goes, she ended up working at the local hospital where she eventually earned a nursing degree. To her credit, she worked 35 years as a full-time nurse while also raising 7 children. Additionally, she was the best grandma ever to 27 grandchildren and too many great-grandchildren to count.

Given her nursing background, when she experienced various symptoms it was only natural for her to ask the doctors with whom she worked for advice. Unfortunately, this lead to several surgeries and a lifetime of prescription medication use. One of those surgeries was a hysterectomy, and some of the prescriptions were hormone replacement medications.

And, although, along with my wife, my mother-in-law was truly the most loving woman I ever met, she struggled with the effects of the hormonal roller coaster, that often accompanies the use of hormone replacement medications, for the rest of her life. To her it was just a "normal" part of her life. However, I think if she were here to tell you, she would have been much happier without the ups and downs. Who do you know that is taking hormone replacement medications and is experiencing similar symptoms? How do you wish to live the rest of your life?

Partial Relief

When a person is suffering, any amount of relief is a good thing. I've been there myself. But, is that where we should stop? It is human nature to 'deal with' whatever is happening until we just can't 'deal with' it anymore. Then, when we do seek care, if we can get enough relief to get us back to where we were, we can 'deal with' the pain again.

I must believe that somewhere down deep everybody would rather have complete relief. Granted, there are a few situations where complete relief is not possible, but in the rest of the situations, complete relief should be the goal. I am constantly amazed by what people put up with. I have had patients that have 'dealt' with this symptom or another for years—some have dealt with them for decades! I have been able to help them, and they were ecstatic.

One patient comes to mind. This lady had been in gymnastics in high school and distinctly remembers falling hard straddling the balance beam. She told me that she could hardly sit down for two weeks after the incident. Within a couple of months, she started having cramping and irregular menstrual cycles. She had found a routine that would get her through her cycle whenever it decided to show up.

This routine included medication and hot baths coupled with hours and hours spent with her laying in the fetal position on her bed. She told me that after the first couple of days it wasn't so bad. The sad part of this story is that this woman was in her early 30's while telling me this story. She had been 'dealing with' these symptoms for 15 years!

After I treated her, she no longer had those chronic symptoms. The last time I saw her, she stated that her cycles were "easy breezy" and that she could actually go about life during those first couple of days without any concerns.

How about you? Have you found a 'routine' that just gets you through? I know that for some women it is hard to believe that they could experience "easy Breezy" menstrual cycles, but with the proper care it is possible.

Sexual Relations

Sexual relations is one of those topics that, if talked about at all, is generally just hinted about without actual conversation. Let's be honest – nobody wants to have a lengthy conversation directed specifically at their intimate relationships. With that said, I must point out that although we don't talk about it, sexual relations with a life's partner is a huge part of the relationship. If sex is taken out of the equation, often people slowly grow apart. Without it, people often end up completely split up.

However, when a woman is experiencing painful, or irregular menstrual cycles, she doesn't often feel like enjoying her partner. I've had patients tell me that intercourse hurt every time even when they weren't on their cycle. Imagine the strain that puts on a relationship. These women wish to please their partners, but they also need to avoid increased pain. It is a situation no one should ever have to be in. There are other conditions that can interfere with one's sexual relations. I once had a patient that had been experiencing endometriosis with very painful cramping. She decided to take her Ob-Gyn's advice and have a hysterectomy.

After the surgery and suggested recovery period, she and her husband decided to make love. To their great dismay, this act caused her immense pain. They decided that perhaps they had been a little too eager to enjoy each other, and decided to give the surgery a couple more weeks to fully heal. However, once again the pain was too unbearable. At this point they felt that something was wrong, and decided to consult her Ob-Gyn. What she found out completely changed her life forever – and not for the better!

As it turns out, her surgeon had been a little too "remove it" happy, and only left her about 2 inches of vaginal depth after her surgery. Her husband, being longer than 2 inches, and used to fully penetrating, was inadvertently causing her pain.

My point in telling you this story is, whoever thinks of sexual relation types of complications from menstrual problems and their common treatments? The title to this chapter is, "**How do you wish to live the rest of your life**". I hope I've broadened your view when you are considering treatment. Hopefully you're thinking about all the potential, life changing, effects. Hopefully you will consider a natural remedy first. You see, if by some remote chance I'm unable to help you, you could still go with the other treatments. However, it you choose my treatment second, I may not be able to help you.

Conditions Worsening with Time

I started this chapter concerned about the effects of doom and gloom. I've tried to keep it rather short for that very reason. However, I have not discussed the fact that conditions never just stay the same. If there is one constant in this world it is the fact that things always change. Life is different now then it was 5 years ago, and 5 years from now it will be a different life again. This holds true for health conditions as well. We humans are either getting healthier or we are getting sicker -- female menstrual disorders included! If you have a disease or irregularity related to your menstrual cycle, it is, also, either getting better or worse.

Human nature directs us to try and ignore the problem and hopefully it will go away. How often do you see that happen? Fact is, people are sometimes beyond help by the time they finally seek the advice of a healthcare provider. If you take the time to look around at the people you know, it won't take long to discover that what I am saying is a fact that we humans all seem to adhere to. It's crazy really!

We all tell a friend or loved one, "you better go have that looked at", but we rarely follow our own advice when it comes to our own health issues. In reality, some conditions do heal themselves, but what about those that just get worse? I would dare say that if a person has a health condition that hasn't healed itself within a couple of weeks or a month, then more than likely it's not going to. I guess you could let it go longer to test my theory, or you could just look around at other people who have 'let it go' and see how they are doing. I am well aware that nobody wants to hear that their condition or disease is going to get worse, but the fact remains that more than likely it will unless proper treatment is administered to intervene.

This concludes this chapter. In the next chapter, I will do my best to dispel the doom and gloom with a few rays of light.

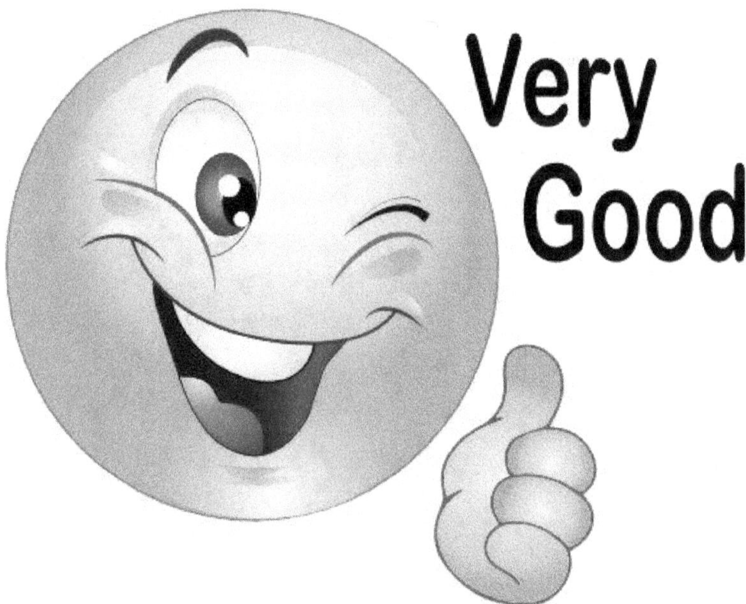

.

Chapter 4: **What If?**

No Medications

At this writing, my wife and I have been married for over 35 years. During that time, she has never been on any type of medication to help regulate her menstrual cycles. There has been a couple of times when her cycles became irregular; however, by working with her body, and looking at all the factors involved, we were able to return her cycles to what is normal for her. She will never need medications to regulate cramping, or to try and keep the timing correct. Her cycles are a little inconvenient as she must keep her feminine products fresh during the days of heavy flow, but other than that, life is just the same during her cycle as it is otherwise.

How does having easy, medication free menstrual cycles sound to you? How would it be to not have a nasty day because you forgot to take your pill(s) that morning?

I recently had a woman come in that was experiencing constant, unexplainable vaginal pain. She has been married for only a few short months, and, although it was not unbearable, the pain was causing some concern in their intimate relations. This patient had been prescribed a pain medication, but decided to visit me instead. She told me just a couple of days ago that it was 'weird' to not have the pain anymore.

Again, I will ask, "How does a medication free life sound to you?"

No Hormonal Medications

How long do you think glands within the body can continue to produce excess hormones before they wear out? What if they do wear out? How long can you, the reader, withstand all the associated symptoms of replacement hormone use? Why would anybody want to find out? These questions and many others are rarely, if ever, asked prior to having a hysterectomy. What if you could avoid a hysterectomy? Think about growing old naturally! As we age, there are many changes that occur throughout the body. Many of those changes are hormone related. Shouldn't we let this amazing organism we call the body change as it needs to with the proper hormones produced and used when and how they are needed? Don't you owe it to yourself, your family, and loved ones to find out if you can live a more natural life without the need for a hysterectomy and hormone replacement medications?

In the next chapter, I will explain a natural treatment that could possibly make the 'no hormone – medication free' life a reality for you. For now, just contemplate the simple ease of such a life style and keep reading.

Complete Relief

How often do people receive care that just makes the pain 'manageable'? I can't tell you how many patients have told me that the medications "take the edge off". Honestly, how often does someone say they had pain then took medication A, B, or C, and "WHA-LA" the pain was gone never to return? It seems to me that have the symptoms completely gone is, and should be, the goal.

A couple of months ago, I had a woman come into my office seeking care for an unrelated matter. As I was speaking with her, she mentioned that I had treated her for menstrual problems 15 years earlier. I vaguely remembered her coming in once she explained to me the situation. None-the less, when I asked her how the treatment 15 years ago had worked, she said, "great!" She had been experiencing normal pain free menstrual cycles ever since. To me, that is how healthcare is supposed to work!

Improved Relations

Is today one of those days when you just don't feel like dealing with people? Let's be downright honest, everybody has those days when they would rather just be alone. Some people have more of those days than others, but, as I said, we all have them. The real question should be, "Is today one of those days because of your menstrual cycle?" Do you find that those days often show up about the same time your cycle does? Wouldn't it be nice if your cycle didn't tend to make you avoid friends and loved ones?

 Don't let me make you feel guilty. The fact is, that when we don't feel good we don't want to be around those that do feel good. If you're one of those ladies that experience bad cramps, or excessive bloating, etc. during your menstrual cycle, then you don't feel good. What if we could decrease or stop those symptoms? Would family relations improve? Would you be able to enjoy your Significant other more?

Do you know other women that seem to never have 'one of those days'? If they are having painless cycles, why couldn't you? I'm telling you that cycles without the drama are possible.

Long Lasting Health

Do you remember when you were just a child? Remember the abundance of energy? Do you remember playing all day and sleeping all night? Do you remember that each day was a new adventure? What happened to those days? Have they been replaced by feeling too achy to even want to get out of bed? Has fighting a headache drained your energy to point of dreading the next adventure? Do you worry about planning a trip because you never know for sure when your next menstrual cycle will start? Are your attempts to get pregnant consuming your life? Wouldn't it be nice to not have to worry about those conditions? Not only that, but wouldn't it be nice to never again have to worry about those problems? Wouldn't it be a wonderful thing to get out of bed each, and every, day knowing it was going to be a good day?

When I first opened my practice, I had a woman come to me that was 86 years old. She was in amazing health. At that time, I X-rayed her entire spine and was in awe at how healthy her vertebral column was. I knew a little about this woman, and knew that her husband's health was not as good. In fact, he was nearly bed ridden. This good woman had worked next to her husband on their family farm for over 60 years. At the time, she was still working next to her husband, but it was to take care of him. She did this herself for about 3 years that I know of. During her care giving efforts, her health remained excellent. In speaking with her, and looking over her health history, I learned that she had always had good health, and that she maintained it with proper diet, enough exercise, and natural early prevention when she felt that something may be awry.

A year or two after I became her treating physician, her husband became too ill for her to take care of at home any longer. Dishearten, she admitted him to an elderly assisted care facility. She went down and spent the entire day with him every day for the next year until he finally passed on. This amazing woman, 89 years old at the time, still in perfect health, drove herself everywhere she needed to go. She still kept her housework up and visited her family. Sadly, when her husband passed, she missed him to the point of truly dying of a broken heart! I was astonished when I learned that she had passed away because I knew that she had been in excellent physical health.

Wouldn't you like this true story to be told of you after a long, loving, healthy life? As I write this, fresh on my memory is my wife's last birthday. She is 6 months younger than I am, and last weekend, for her birthday, she wanted to go camping and do some hiking. We drove to a mountain camping area that we are fond of and set up camp. It had rained that afternoon, but the evening was beautiful. She felt like going for a little walk, so we headed up the canyon. The next morning, we were curious how far we had walked the evening before. We learned, after driving the same route, that we had walked about 6 miles. Now remember, this was in the mountains at about 8,000 feet of elevation.

Now, I understand most, if not all of you reading this could go walk 6 miles. I have a couple of questions for you though, 1) Do you just go walk 6 miles because you feel like going for a walk? 2) How do you feel the next day?

After we completed our 6-mile walk, we were back at camp roasting hot dogs and playing games. The next morning, we put on our backpacks and completed another 6 miles on a mountain trail next to a beautiful river. On this hike, we gained considerable elevation before returning to camp.

Again, I am aware that to many of you reading this it doesn't seem like a big deal. However, I've been practicing for 20 years, and I can tell you that the greatest majority of people in their mid-50's don't just go for a 6-mile walk. And, if they do, they don't get up the next morning and hike uphill for another 6 miles with a backpack on their backs.

What if you could enjoy life like the older lady I told you about? What if you could go hiking at 50 or 60 years old like no big deal? It's possible! You just need to decide and then take the appropriate actions to achieve your desired outcome.

Chapter 5: THE ANSWER (NATURAL TREATMENT)

Anatomy

Now don't let the title of this section scare you! I remember when I was going to school the thought of anatomy class would strike un-told horrors in the minds of many aspiring students. This will not be the case in this section; however, I must lay some ground work of how the human body works before explaining how and why my natural treatment works.

To start off, I will start at the top – literally! The top for our purposes is the head, or, more specifically, the brain. The brain is in total control of our entire bodies. If you think about it, no other organ is completely incased in bone. Some organs are fairly well protected, but not like our brains. This protection is because our master controller (our brain) has such an important function. Our brains are made up of billions of specialized cells we call nerve bodies. These nerve bodies have thin, finger-like extensions on them that reach out to other nerve bodies for communication purposes. Additionally, some of these extensions must communicate with other parts of the body. These extensions form together and become the spinal cord and spinal nerves. By utilizing the nerves throughout our bodies, the brain is able to both gather information and send commands to and from whatever the end organ in our body is. This communication system in whole is called the nervous system, and if it is working at optimal levels we are healthy. Through the nervous system, the brain can manage the functions of our entire bodies – including all the menstrual organs and glands and their functions.

There, also, exists some anatomical structures designed to help the nervous system work at that optimal level mentioned. One of these structures is the spinal, or vertebral, column. The spinal column is really an amazing structure. It is designed to protect the spinal cord with nearly complete bony encasement, yet allow nerves to exit the spinal canal without impediment. Inside the spinal column is the spinal canal. The spinal cord descends within the canal, but is surrounded by a tough, almost canvas like pouch called the thecal sac. The thecal sac allows the spinal cord to move as needed, but also channels the fluid we call cerebral spinal fluid to flow down and around the spinal cord. At each vertebral level, nerves exit the spinal cord. In order to exit, the nerves must first pierce the thecal sac then proceed out the little holes that are in between the vertebra. Where this occurs, the thecal sac protrudes outward a short distance with the nerve. If you were to dissect the thecal sac, it would be shaped kind of like a long leaf with pointed edges where the nerves exit. These outward projections play a role in menstrual health, and I will discuss them in more detail later.

Other structures include ligaments which position the nerves and keep them in their proper position during movement. One such ligament, that plays an important role, is called the Ligamentous terminalis. Think of this ligament as the anchoring ligament. The anchoring ligament attaches to the very bottom part of the spinal cord and goes down through the pelvis and attaches to the tailbone. The purpose of this ligament is to keep the proper tension on the spinal cord during movement. I will discuss the importance of this ligament in greater detail later in the book.

Finally, various joints on the vertebral column allow for the great amount of motion that we humans enjoy. There are, obviously, other structures, but for our purposes, this general description will do.

At the bottom of our spinal column is the supporting structure we call the pelvis. The pelvis acts like a foundation for our spine, and creates stability as we move about our world. The pelvis includes 4 bones. Two of these bones (one right and one left) are the bones we can feel on our sides directly above our legs. The other two are directly below the vertebral column in the back. The upper bone is an inverted wedge-shaped bone that supports our vertebral column and disperses the weight out to the first two bones and on to our legs. The lower of these two bones is the small bone at the very bottom that we call the tailbone. The anchoring ligament attaches here. Our tailbone plays a very important, but largely overlooked, role in female menstrual health. I will discuss this role a little later.

What the reader needs to get from the above explanation is an overall picture of how the brain connects to the spinal cord which travels down the spinal canal. One also needs to envision the nerves that exit the spinal column at each vertebral level to create a communication network throughout the entire body. Also, an understanding of the various ligaments, including the anchoring ligament, that keep the spinal cord centered within the spinal canal should be gained. Please understand that this description is and over-simplification of the anatomy in question, but creates a good starting point for the next few sections.

Physiology

Again, the title of this section can be intimidating, but all it really means is how the anatomical structures discussed interact with each other. If we look at our cars, we see the various parts such as the doors, tires, bumpers, headlights, seats, steering wheel, engine, transmission, etc. These parts, or structures, that make up the overall car are the car's "anatomy." Now, if we think about how each of the structures, or parts, work together to create transportation, that would be the "physiology" of the car. For example, in order to pull out onto the street, one must start the engine; which turns the transmission; which rotates the tires; which starts the car moving forward. Additionally, we must turn the steering wheel which angles the tires; which guides the car to where we want it to go. The same principle is true with the relationship between the anatomy of the human body and the physiology of the body.

In this brief description, I will again just hit the highlights of the physiology in question. Please keep in mind that the complexity of a complete explanation is beyond the scope of this book.

Starting again at the top, the brain monitors and controls the function of our bodies. This is accomplished by electrical impulses (that I will call nerve impulses) being transmitted along the nerves. Monitoring information is initiated somewhere out in the body and causes a nerve impulse to be started and transmitted along the nerve, into the spinal cord, and up to the brain. The brain gathers all the monitoring information, and uses it to generate command signals which become nerve impulses that travel back down the spinal cord. From the spinal cord, the impulses exit via the nerves. Upon reaching the targeted organ, the impulse causes the wanted response to keep the body healthy and functioning. A good example of the monitoring/command impulse cycle would be when you touch something very hot. First, the information creates many impulses in the sensory receptors in your skin. These impulses travel from the receptors to the connected nerves, into the spinal cord, and up to the brain. Your brain generates multiple command impulses that travel down the cord, out the nerves, and onto the many muscles responsible to quickly move your hand away.

The above simple example works in every function of our bodies. The nerve impulses don't have to be something changing or dangerous as the example would indicate. The brain receives and creates billions of impulses every minute. Generally, this looks more like the sensory organ sending an impulse that says, "everything is A-Okay." The brain then responds with an impulse that says, "great, keep up the good work." This constant communication is how we maintain our health. If, for some reason, the end organ sends an impulse to the brain that says, "hey, I have a problem," then the brain will make a decision based on all the monitoring data, and send a response impulse back to tell the body how to react. If the body, because of some outside condition, can't react as the brain instructs then we become unhealthy.

There are, as discussed, supporting structures that allow the nerve impulses to travel properly. As you can imagine, when we move about our world many different forces act upon our bodies. Some of these forces are of interest when it comes to proper nerve function. One such force is created when we bend over and stand back up. Can you picture how the back portion of your spine would stretch and the front portion would compress when you bend over?

Well, the spinal cord is in the back portion of the spine, therefore, as we bend, the cord is stretched. When we stand again, the stretch is released. If this were to happen repeatedly, without the various supporting structures to hold the cord in its proper place, the cord could 'bunch up' within the canal. One of the main supporting structures which keeps the cord from bunching up, is the anchoring ligament. The anchoring ligament holds tension on the cord to pull it back down when it is stretched up. There are other ligaments higher in the canal that connect the cord to the thecal sac and the thecal sac to the vertebra. These ligaments will not be discussed in this work. Let it suffice to know that they exist. Finally, there are many such structures along the many paths of the nerves that perform similar functions. The anchoring ligament can affect women's menstrual health and is, therefore, mentioned here.

In the last section, I briefly mentioned the fluid that our spinal cords are immersed in. This fluid is called cerebral spinal fluid. I must make a quick comment about this life sustaining fluid. Cerebral spinal fluid has a few different functions; however, for this discussion, I only need to explain one of those functions. First off, cerebral spinal fluid is produced in the central part of the brain, and flows down the thecal sac bathing the spinal cord and exiting nerves as it goes. This flow brings with it the nutrients and oxygen that the cord and nerves need to remain healthy and functioning. If for some reason the fluid is blocked in its flow, or not able to fully bath the spinal cord and nerves, then those nerves are slowly starved of vital nutrients and oxygen. This decrease in nutrients and oxygen can, and often does, lead to an unhealthy state. Again, I will expound on this in a later section.

There is one other condition in general terms that I must touch upon. Do you recall, in an earlier chapter, I talked about the mechanic saying he could un-plug the check engine light? Well, along that same train of thought, what if something interrupts the flow of nerve impulses to and from the brain? What happens if the brain doesn't receive the monitoring information? Or, what happens if the end organ doesn't receive the command impulses? In the example at the beginning of this section, if the brain didn't receive the information about the very hot object, our hand would be badly burned.

The same is true if the muscles used to move the hand away didn't receive the command impulses from the brain. I know this seems like a simple example; however, this is an important concept that I will expand upon in the next sections. I will also discuss how the nerve impulses can be, and often are, interrupted.

The Problem

Good, you've read to this point. That means you made it through the somewhat tedious explanation of the anatomy and physiology. It is difficult to give enough detail without giving too much. Stay with me and I will tie it all together.

As the title of this section implies, my goal is to explain a problem that many ladies with menstrual cycle dysfunction have. This problem is very often overlooked at best, and not even know about most commonly. If you will recall, I briefly mentioned the cerebral spinal fluid a couple of times. I discussed how it is supposed to bath the spinal cord and the exiting nerves. This bathing flow is accomplished, in great part, by the motion of our bodies as we breathe. You see, when we inhale our spine slightly straightens and out head slightly enlarges.

This causes our brain to travel with our head in an upward direction. Please keep in mind that I'm not talking about a huge change in position. The upward movement, along with the swelling of the head and straightening of the spine, is very slight. None-the-less, this combination of action when we inhale causes the tension on the cord to slightly increase which causes the tension on all the exiting nerves to slightly increase. The increased tension is kept in check by the anchoring ligament; however, the same tension causes all the exiting nerves to be pulled back into the spinal canal just a little bit.

When we exhale, the spine returns to its beginning position. The head slightly shrinks, and the tension is released from the cord and nerves. The decreased tension allows the nerves to once again reposition out of the spinal canal. At this point we generally inhale again and the whole action repeats.

The thing I need you to understand is that when the exiting nerves move in and out of the canal, the motion creates a rhythmic flow of the cerebral spinal fluid around the exiting portion of the nerves. If the nerves are not allowed to move in and out, then the cerebral spinal fluid will pool in the pointed projections of the thecal sac where the nerves exit. This pooling causes a stagnation, if you will, of the cerebral spinal fluid at that point. It is kind of like how water in a creek will pool in the wide spot along the bank, and create an eddy. The water in the main part of the creek is still flowing nicely, but in the eddy the water is somewhat stagnant. (Read this paragraph again – its important!)

This stagnation of cerebral spinal fluid causes the nerve to be somewhat starved of vital nutrients and oxygen. Without the proper nutrition, the nerve can't transmit the nerve impulse efficiently which doesn't allow the brain to receive all the needed information to create proper command impulses.

I realize this explanation is becoming somewhat lengthy, but bear with me. We are heading down the home straight – I promise.

The obvious question at this point is, "what would stop the normal motion of the nerves moving in and out of the canal as we breathe?" Existing are a few different answers to that question; however, for the purposes of this book, I will discuss only two.

The first has to do with the anchoring ligament. If tension in the anchoring ligament is increased, then it will pull down on the thecal sac and, in turn, the spinal cord. With increased tension pulling down, any upward tension, as we bend or inhale, will not be enough to allow the nerves to move into the canal properly. Thus, the rhythmic flow of cerebral spinal fluid is slowed, or stopped, and the nerves become malnourished. A common way for the tension on the anchoring ligament to increase is by the tailbone repositioning in such a way as to move the anchoring point further from the canal. This is most commonly accomplished by the tailbone being tilted inward.

All structures that make up the anatomy of the human body have a proper position and function. The same is true for the tailbone. As with other anatomical structures, if moved from proper position, the tailbone can cause dysfunction. I will discuss the outside influences that can cause this inward displacement in the next section.

Before discussing the second cause of the nerves not moving normally, there is one other aspect of the over-tensioned anchoring ligament that I need to point out. Our spinal cord, and our thecal sac, and all the other structures discussed are comprised of living tissue. What this means is that it is not rigid. Living tissue has a certain amount of normal plasticity. This allows for a little bit of stretch to occur in all our tissues. I alluded to this when I talked about the stretch that occurs when we bend over.

The spinal cord and nerves, also, have the ability to stretch somewhat. Because of this stretch, the nerves at the lower end of the spinal cord are affected by the tension in the anchoring ligament more than the nerves in the upper portion of the cord. As it so happens, the nerves in the lower part of the cord are the nerves that go to the reproductive organs. Thus, increased tension on the nerves of the lower cord can cause reproductive, or menstrual cycle irregularities for a female. That said, we must allow for the fact that we are all unique. Increased tension in the cord for some people only affects the lower nerves, while increased tension for others can affect the upper nerves as well. For example, increased tension on the anchoring ligament can cause headaches. The spinal cord is an extension of the brain. If you pull on the cord, you must also pull on the brain.

The second cause, that I will discuss, of the nerves not moving in and out of the canal properly concerns the structures surrounding the exiting nerve itself. The entire concept of the nerves freely moving in and out of the canal is based on there being no friction on the nerves as they attempt to move. What if something in or around the hole where the nerve exits the vertebral column puts pressure on the nerve? This pressure could cause, for lack of a better word, a pinching type action to hold the nerve from moving. In addition to the reduction in motion, this pressure could also impede the normal transmission of the nerve impulses.

One way to increase the pressure on the nerves where they exit, is if the joints near the exiting holes become inflamed and swollen. The swelling will push into the region reserved for the exiting nerve and produce the increased pressure described. As you can imagine, increasing pressure on the nerve while at the same time reducing its vital nutrition and oxygen because of cerebral spinal fluid pooling, will interrupt the communication between the body and the brain.

In an earlier section, I talked about the wires that carry the internet signal to a building being interrupted. In that instance, I was explaining the hormones that flow throughout the body. Well, if the nerve with increased pressure spoken about above is one that communicates with a gland that produces hormones, then the body's hormonal WIFI will be affected. Taking it one step further, if that gland helps regulate the hormones involved with the menstrual cycle, then the menstrual cycle becomes irregular.

I truly hope that you, the reader, have gotten a basic understanding of the anatomy and physiology that I've described. I also hope that you can see a couple of the possible complications I've attempted to explain. In the next section, I will give a few examples of how the increased tension in the anchoring ligament occurs along with a few examples of how the vertebral joints become inflamed and swollen.

How It Happened

Surely if you've read to this point, you must be wondering if one or more of the conditions described apply to you. I'm going to talk about a few possibilities of how you may have acquired one or more of these conditions. Once again, it is next to impossible to cover every scenario in this writing. I encourage you to think about your own life's experiences to see if something similar may have happened to you.

I would dare say that the most common way for the tailbone to be mal-positioned forward is by some sort of injury. Often, the injury is minimized in the mind of the injured. For example, as a child, a girl will land in a seated position on the frame of a trampoline, and experience pain in the tailbone region for a few days. Once the pain goes away, the incident is forgotten. Additionally, that type of injury and associated pain can be somewhat embarrassing for a young girl to talk about, so when the pain goes away she is relieved.

Similar injuries can occur by wrecking a bicycle, or in gymnastics. Sometimes riding a horse, especially bareback, can cause the tailbone to be displaced forward. I have had some ladies that remembered slipping on ice, and falling on the stairs or sidewalk in a seated position. Another common injury occurs just from extended time sitting. In our society, many women have careers that require many hours in front of a computer screen. When we get tired, our muscle tone decreases, and for some women that leaves them sitting directly on their tailbones for hours day after day. There are as many types of accidents as there are different types of people and places. I think you get the idea with what I've discussed.

Another method by which the tailbone can be moved forward is by physical abuse. The abuse can be anywhere from playfully rough housing to physically abusive relationships. I had one young woman come to me, that said when she was in junior high school it was a game with her friends to sneak up and kick each other playfully in the bottom. This particular young lady recalled being kicked a little too hard a couple of times. Unfortunately, this same type of injury occurs all too often in physically abusive adult relationships.

One last injury method before moving on to other ways the tailbone can be displaced forward. I had a woman tell me one time that she felt her husband was the cause of her problem. Apparently, he was a long-haul trucker, and would be gone all week on the road. When he would get home, they liked to enjoy their marital rights on her workbench. She would bend forward over the bench and they would make love with him behind her. She said that occasionally she felt like he was hitting directly on her tailbone with his pubic region.

There are other ways that the tailbone can be displaced forward that don't involve direct injury. One very common way, in our society, is stress. When I was in school, a study was released that credited stress with decreasing a person's life span by as much as 30 years. I was hesitant to believe these findings. Then, shortly after I graduated, a man I was close to passed away. This man had lived a very stressful lifestyle, and passed away at only 56 years old. The reason I bring this up is because his siblings lived into their 80's and 90's. In fact, one of his older siblings is still alive as of this writing.

Stress can cause many unhealthy conditions in our bodies. We commonly think of the heart problems, or the digestion problems associated with stress. However, stress can affect every system of our bodies. The list is too lengthy to cover in this book, but I can tell you that many of the patients I see have health issues directly related to stress. This definitely includes patients with menstrual health issues. I have tried to understand just exactly how the stress causes the tailbone to move forward, but, honestly, have yet to make a defined connection. I believe it is hard to pin down exactly because stress affect everybody differently. What I can tell you is, that by moving the tailbone back to a more normal position, these patients experience relief.

One last possibility before I move on to the next section. This last method is closely related to stress, but is important enough that it deserves its own discussion. The topic is diet. We live in a world where, even if we try, it is hard to have a healthy diet. There is new research being published continuously about this growing problem. The fact is, that feeding the world is really quiet a challenge in and of itself. Healthfully feeding the world is an entirely greater challenge. If we add stress and time demands into the picture, then our food quality choices really head towards the bottom of the healthy food list.
 It is sort of sad really. We know that eating poor quality food causes disease, but we do it anyway! This is such an epidemic, that many people totally avoid "healthy" food because it doesn't taste good to

them. None-the-less, our bodies need the basic building blocks of nutrition in order to be healthy. Without these essential building blocks, we become sick.

By eating poor quality food, our bodies want more food. Basically, we are hungry more often. This is because our bodies are trying to get the nutrients it needs to function properly. By eating more of the same nutrient poor food, we struggle with weight gain. Our bodies are efficient, and we store the excess of the nutrients we are getting while attempting to get the nutrients we lack. With increased weight, and lack of proper nutrition and exercise, we feel less energetic. This decrease in energy leads to a more sedentary lifestyle which encourages snacking on unhealthy foods. An increase in weight and decrease in energy leads to poor posture as well. The changes in the way gravity acts upon the human frame due to poor posture can cause abnormal alignment of various bones. This includes the tailbone. Again, I can tell you that it has been my experience, that by repositioning the tailbone to a more normal position, ladies see an improvement in both menstrual irregularities and in energy. I have even had some ladies tell me they have lost weight after the procedure. I had one lady that requested I reposition her tailbone 3 times because she lost 8 to 10 pounds each time.

Thus far in this section I have only discussed ways the tailbone can become displaced forward. If you recall from the previous section, I also mentioned the nerves themselves being affected by a pinching type pressure where they exit the vertebral column. I also promised to discuss a few examples of how that could happen. These examples fall into 3 categories. The categories parallel the conditions already discussed for the tailbone. The three categories are thoughts, traumas, and toxins.

In our society, these can be closely converted to stress, injury, and poor diet. I will not repeat the conversations about stress and diet as they affect the entire body, and you, the reader, should easily be able to expand the previous discussions to include the entire spine. I will, however, discuss a little bit about traumas or injuries.

Imagine how much force our bodies absorb when we fall. Or, the force involved with an automobile accident. Luckily, we are designed to withstand a certain degree of impact, but that doesn't mean we don't sustain injuries from those impacts. Often the injury is what we consider minor. We have all experienced being hurt, and a few days later the pain is gone.

My question to you is, "just because the pain is gone, does that mean the injury is fully healed?" Does the absence of pain indicate health? It is human nature to believe that yes will answer both questions asked. However, most often, this is not the case. Research shows that it can take years to heal certain injuries, if they heal at all. This is common in the vertebral column. Can you see that the forces associated with any impact must be absorbed throughout the body? Try this experiment. First, walk up to within two or three inches of a wall, or door frame, etc. Now, try to feel what your entire body is doing while you carefully, and easily, slightly fall into a leaning position onto the wall. Did you feel the impact in your legs? It may not have been much, but you should have been able to feel it. Did you feel it in your spine? What about your head and neck? What if the impact were much greater than in our little experiment? Would it be possible that injury could have occurred to your vertebra that didn't quickly heal?

The reality is that injury can, and does, occur. Very commonly this injury is to the joints of the spine and they become inflamed and swollen as described in the last section. Additionally, unless something is done to allow these joints to properly heal, they can stay inflamed for long periods of time – even years! This means that the nerves could have pressure on them for years. This also means that the person could be symptomatic, in one way or another, for years. How long have you been experiencing menstrual health issues? Did you experience an injury prior to the menstrual health issues starting? It is important that you understand that the inflamed joints on the vertebral column may not be painful, but can still be swollen and affecting the exiting nerves.

The above discussion should have given you an understanding of how unhealthy conditions occur. The actual concern, however, should be how do correct the problem. How to move the tailbone back into a more normal position, and how reduce the inflammation and swelling in the vertebral joints. That will be the topic of the next section.

How Do We Fix It?

The treatment to move the tailbone back into a more normal position is a rather simple procedure for the doctor; however, for the patient it can sometimes be a little intimidating. You see, the tailbone is at the very bottom of the spine or pelvis. It is also somewhat surrounded by the layers of gluteal muscles. This makes it difficult to access. The best way to gain access is for the doctor to gently insert his or her index finger into the anal opening, which is directly below the tailbone, and apply just enough outward pressure to move the tailbone to that more normal position mentioned. The intimidating part for some women is the thought of first getting undressed, and second having someone digitally penetrate their anal opening. I want to put any worries at this point to rest.

In my office, when a woman is to be treated, she is taken to a room and allowed to change into a gown which opens to the back. She is then instructed to wrap a towel around her waist with the towel covering the back of the gown. In this way, she is completely covered, and her integrity is preserved.

When I start the procedure, I have the patient lie face down with a cushion or bolster under her waist. Then I lift the towel just enough to make sure I'm in the right place. Using my gloved index finger, I apply just enough lubricant to allow as easy of an entry as possible. Once I've verified the correct position and applied the lubricant, I again cover the patient with the towel. At this point, I should explain that my index finger is generally smaller in diameter than the exiting fecal matter when we defecate, therefore, the greatest majority of women tell me the procedure was a lot easier for them than they expected. After completing the treatment, I leave the room to give the patient time to clean up and re-dress.

In all the years that I have been treating patients, I have discovered that most women are so sick and tired of the symptoms they are experiencing that this sometimes-intimidating procedure, to start them on the healing path, is not that big of a deal. With that said, I have had a few ladies that couldn't bring themselves to have the treatment. What is interesting about that is the fact that a great percentage of those ladies return at a later date and have the treatment anyway. All I can say is it works! Women get tremendous relief from their menstrual irregularities after treatment.

In addition to repositioning the tailbone, we need to relieve any pressure that may be restricting any of the exiting nerves in the vertebral column. This is done through a chiropractic adjustment. Often people will say they are, "out of place." This is not completely accurate. Being out of motion is a more accurate description. You see, joints are designed to allow motion in the body. If that motion is restricted or stopped, then the joint becomes inflamed and swollen. Through the proper delivery of a specific chiropractic adjustment, the joints can be put back into normal motion.

In my office, after adjusting the tailbone back into a more normal position, I check the rest of the patient's spine, and adjust any vertebra that may have decreased normal motion. By doing this, the healing process is allowed to begin. After the adjustment, I usually recommend the patient uses ice to further help reduce the swelling. Additionally, I recommend the patient returns to my office within 24 to 48 hours for a follow up treatment. On this second visit, I only adjust the spine.

I have found, through years of experience, that the patient healing process requires 3 such visits each week for 2 to 4 weeks. I only adjust the spine in most of these visits. On the first visit of the second week, however, I adjust the tailbone again as a precautionary procedure. I have found that many women need the second repositioning of the tailbone to fully gain the benefits sought. By following this schedule, patients see a very high percentage of improvement.

In the next chapter, I will expound upon the specifics of the described treatment, so keep reading!
Have You Heard of This Treatment? Why Not?

About a month ago, I had a patient tell me that her aunt had told her about the tailbone repositioning treatment, and that she was excited to get hers treated. This patient's aunt had a positive experience, and had suggested she also have the procedure. I treated her, and she, too, had a positive response.
 I tell you this story because this particular patient is one of only a very small group that has actually heard of having their tailbone adjusted. Very few women in the general population know that having their tailbone repositioned can help with menstrual cycle irregularities and the associated symptoms.

I believe the knowledge of this potentially life changing treatment is little known because of a variety of reasons. To start with, we live in a society where most people seek the care and advice of a medical doctor when they are experiencing symptoms. When it comes to repositioning the tailbone, most, if not all, medical doctors and Ob-Gyns are never taught the specifics of the treatment. Therefore, they cannot perform a procedure that they are unaware of.

Secondly, due to the sensitive nature of the treatment, many chiropractors shy away from performing the internal tailbone (or coccyx) adjustment. We live in such a litigious society that I can't really blame them. I have always found that if I explain to the patient what I recommend, and give them the choice of the care, I never have any concerns. I have been working with patients, and doing tailbone adjustments, for twenty years and have never even be threatened with a law suit. I earnestly believe that this procedure has, and still can, help thousands, or tens of thousands, of women suffering from menstrual related symptoms; therefore, I still recommend and perform internal coccyx adjustments in my office. In fact, there is such a demand for this treatment that I am specializing in just these types of cases.

Lastly, and unfortunately, most healthcare providers are so busy taking care of patients with other conditions that they just don't have the time required to add internal coccyx adjustments to their schedule. I have always, and will always, tried to do what is best for the patient. If a woman presents in my office with menstrual related symptoms, I at least tell her about the possible treatment options, and give her the information with which to make an educated decision for her care. I feel as though I would be negligent in my duties as a healthcare provider if I did not.

What about you? Have you ever heard of the internal tailbone (coccyx) adjusting procedure? As you sit there reading this are you thinking, "is this for real?" Are you wondering, "is this Fitzgerald guy for real?" If you are I completely understand. My suggestion is that you don't just take my word for it. Do some research—check me out! I am confident that you will find I am leading you in the right direction. I realize at this point you probably still have questions. That is why in the next chapter I will explain in a little depth how and why this treatment works.

Chapter 6: **How and Why it Works**

Physiology

I believe that the reason, when I was in school, that many students feared physiology was because there is so much to it. None of the actual physiology is hard in and of itself. However, when a person looks at the shear volumes of information about the subject it becomes intimidating. Don't let that happen to you. I am going to recap just a little as I explain how our bodies benefit from being adjusted, and why the tail bone adjustment works.

I hope you have a somewhat clear picture in your head of the anatomy of our spines. Remember I described the nerve cell extensions coming from the brain and gathering together to form the spinal cord? As these cell extensions group together, they form what we refer to as a nerve. These nerves exit the spinal canal through the holes formed between the vertebra at each level in order to communicate with the entire body. Additionally, I told you about the thecal sac which encloses the cord, and allows the cerebral spinal fluid to flow around the cord. I also described how the anchoring ligament attaches to the bottom of the spinal cord, and goes down to the back, top of the tailbone. Finely, I explained joints that are located between the vertebra and close to the exiting nerves.

If you have a clear picture of the structures in the previous paragraph, then it should be a simple step to see how the tailbone adjustment works. If you remember, I described a few ways that the tailbone can be pushed forward. Can you see that if the tailbone is re-positioned back to a more normal position then it will relieve the extra tension off of the anchoring ligament? Relieving the extra tension will, in turn, reduce the tension on the spinal cord.

Remember how I explained that the exiting nerves normally move out and back in to the spinal canal as we move and breathe? Well, by reducing the tension on the spinal cord, the nerves are allowed to move more normally. Again, that more normal motion creates a rhythmic flow of the cerebral spinal fluid around the cord and exiting nerves. This flow bathes the exiting nerve right at the point where it exits the thecal sac. This rhythmic flow allows the exiting nerve to be fully nourished and fully oxygenated. A fully nourished and oxygenated nerve is a healthy, functioning nerve which means it will transmit the nerve impulses with efficiency. This proper transmission of nerve impulses allows the brain to fully communicate with the body and to start the healing process.

For purposes of this discussion, I must again point out that the nerves and spinal cord are living tissue. Inherent in living tissue is a certain amount of pliability. Because of this pliability, the lower portion of the spinal cord is generally the most affected by extra tension from a forward displaced tailbone. The upper portion of the cord has greater notion because it is further away from the anchoring ligament, and, thus, benefits from the pliability over a greater distance. To complete this section, I will briefly mention that the reason the re-positioning of the tailbone helps with menstrual cycle disorders is because the lowest nerves on the spinal cord are the ones that connect the reproductive organs to the brain. Therefore, by reducing the tension on the anchoring ligament, the brain can again communicate with the reproductive organs, including the uterus, and begin to monitor and regulate the function of these organs. When properly regulated, the reproductive organs are healthy and function properly.

Ice

Toward the end of the last chapter, I quickly mentioned having the patient use ice. I decided to wait and explain more about the use of ice in this chapter as how and why the treatment works is the topic at hand. Additionally, using ice is more closely related to the joints that are located by the exiting nerves. If you recall, I talked about the joints between the vertebra becoming inflamed. It is this inflammation that responds best to ice.

In order to fully explain this, I must first explain how the joints become inflamed. As you can imagine, all joints in the human body are primarily designed for motion. This motion is created when the joint surface on one bone is made to slide across the joint surface of the adjacent bone. Within the small space between the two joint surfaces is a fluid that, much like the cerebral spinal fluid, brings the nutrition and oxygen to the cells that form the joint surfaces. This same fluid is also responsible to carry away the metabolic waste that is created once the nutrition and oxygen is consumed by the cells (this fluid has other functions as well, but will not be discussed in this book.)

If you recall, in an earlier chapter, I gave a few examples of how we can become unhealthy. I explained injury, and talked about stress and poor diet. Well, through those various ways, the joints of the spine can be affected and not allow normal motion at that vertebral level. The normal motion acts somewhat like a pump to help keep the oxygenated, nutrient rich fluid flowing through the joint space. If the joint experiences reduced or complete loss of normal motion, then the fluid does not flow properly. However, the cells in the joint space continue to consume oxygen and nutrition, so metabolic waste continues to be generated. Without proper flow, the waste builds up and becomes an irritant to the cells. Our bodies respond by sending more fluid to the area by way of increased blood flow. Blood brings with it the substances used in healing; however, without proper joint motion those healing substances have a difficult time getting into the joint space. Therefore, the area just becomes more inflamed with more swelling. As discussed earlier, the only place for this extra swelling to expand is into the space reserved for the exiting nerves. Thus, the nerve impulse in that nerve is affected, and our bodies move away from optimum health.

By putting the normal motion back into the joint with a chiropractic adjustment, the root cause of the symptoms is being addressed. However, the swelling and inflammation must also be addressed. This is where the ice comes into play. Our bodies respond to inflammation by adding heat to the area. Ice helps reduce that heat. Our bodies also cause the blood vessels in the area to dilate to increase the blood flow discussed. Ice causes our blood vessels to constrict which reduces the flow of fluid into the tissues. Finally, the ice does not slow the flow of the fluid from the joint space and into the lymph system which is responsible to carry the excess away. With these functions in mind, lets discuss the correct procedure with which to use ice for the best results.

It is common in our society to do whatever is easiest. Therefore, we have at our disposal various types of frozen objects. The most common of these objects is a freezer gel pack. I would advise you at this point to not use them. I will explain why a little later. The fact is, I would advise you to not use any of the convenient cooling objects such as, frozen vegetables, blue ice, freezer gel packs, or frozen rice bags to name a few.

The best way to use ice is to use ICE! Yes, frozen water ice! My recommendation is to put about 1½ inches of liquid water in the bottom of a gallon sized freezer storage bag. You know, the ones that snap together along the top to seal and lock the bag closed. Then add about an ice cube tray full of frozen water ice. When you use this bag of ice water on the affected area, put it directly on the skin. Yes, I know that it is cold! I will explain why in just a bit. Anyway, put the plastic bag right against the skin without a towel or clothing to insulate it. Leave the ice on until the affected area goes numb. It will take approximately 15 minutes for the numbness to occur, but it is the numb feeling that signals removal of the ice – not the 15 minutes passing on the clock. It may only take 13 minutes, or it may take 18 minutes to go numb as everybody is a little different. None-the-less, once numb, remove the bag. Leave the ice off for at least 2 hours before re-applying ice again for the next treatment.

Why do I advise using ice in this manner? Allow me to elaborate. When frozen water ice and liquid water are mixed, the resulting solution is always 32oF as long as there is still ice and water together. 32oF will not freeze the skin. It may feel frozen, but it is just very cold. Additionally, the solution will stay 32oF until all the ice is melted. Lastly, ice and water is the only mixture to behave that way. Because ice and water is the only solution to stay at 32oF, none of the other items mentioned will perform the same. All of the ice replacement items start out too cold and warm up too quickly. Therefore, the body doesn't fully get the benefit of the ice treatment like it does with ice and water as described.

I recommend using the ice 4 times a day for 2 to 4 days following injury. Don't despair if you haven't been using ice as you can start now. I have had many patients that once I got them off the heat and using ice, they healed very well. I usually tell patients to use the ice at breakfast time, at lunch time, at dinner time, and just before going to bed at night. The only other requirement is to wait at least 2 hours from the time they remove the ice before re-applying it to the same area. If a person is in a lot of pain, then the ice could be used more than 4 times per day, but, remember, always wait at least 2 hours in between removing and re-applying.

As a last note for this section, I would warn you to not – I repeat, do not – use heat in any way shape or form on an injury. I am well aware that many healthcare professionals recommend using heat because it feel good. I am telling you, here and now, don't do it! If you recall from my earlier discussion, the body dilates the blood vessels in the injury area. Additionally, there is heat involved as the area becomes inflamed. Applying heat to the skin does the same things. Applying heat adds more heat and further dilates the blood vessels which, ultimately, leads to more inflammation. Basically, applied heat makes the injury worse in the long run. I recommend you fore go the short term "feel good" of heat for the long-term healing of ice.

The Body's Ability to Heal Itself

When I first opened my practice, many years ago, I had a woman present to me with severe low back pain, severe upper back pain, and severe cramping during her menstrual cycle. Additionally, she was experiencing totally irregular timing on her cycles. As I spoke with her, she mentioned that she slept with her low back on a heating pad every night. Further, she had a second heating pad by her bed that she would put on her lower abdomen when the cramps were particularly bad. We had the conversation about heat found in the previous section, and I advised her to use ice. She disagreed with me, and continued to use the heat. She told me that there was no way she would be able to sleep without her heating pad. As I worked with her, the topic became somewhat of a humorous challenge between us. I would smile and ask if she had tried the ice yet, and she would smile back and ask if I had tried the heat yet. If I remember correctly, we went back and forth on the ice/heat dilemma for a couple of months. Then one day she told me that she had gone on a trip and forgotten to pack her heating pad. While at the hotel, she finally gave in and decide to try the ice treatment.

Now, as you can imagine, I wouldn't be telling this story if it hadn't worked. The fact is, she began to feel so much better that her frequency of visits at my office greatly reduced. She put her heating pads in storage, and became a raving fan of the ice. As far as I know, she hasn't used the heat once since that time. The interesting thing about this story is that she had slept on that heating pad for years. For years she was in pain. For years she felt she had to live with the pain. For years none of the other healthcare professionals could figure out what was causing her to be unhealthy. Once I started treating the cause of the symptoms, and giving her body the proper opportunity to heal, she dramatically improved. In fact, she healed so quickly I was even a little surprised.

The same is true for all humans. Given the proper opportunity, we all have this amazing healing power within us. Unless we have become so ill that the body's healing power is totally overcome, we can heal. Yes – read that again – We Can Heal!! Obviously, there are disease processes that can overcome this amazing healing power in which case the outcome is often grime. But, even in some of those cases the body heals.

I am constantly amazed when a patient tells me that they've had one symptom or another for so long that there is nothing I can do for it. I generally remind the patient of the body's fantastic innate ability to heal itself, and recommend a care regiment. Usually, if the patient will follow my recommendations, we see success. I have helped so many of these types of patients that it is just "old hat" now when they tell me how much better they are doing. In fact, if a patient doesn't respond as expected, I am genuinely surprised.

My entire job as a healthcare provider is to give the body the proper opportunity to heal itself. That statement may make it sound overly simple, but the secret is in knowing how to give the body that opportunity. I have been doing that very thing for so long now, and seen so many patients, that rarely do I get stumped on how to help someone.

Some years ago, I had a woman seek my care because she had been experiencing headaches for over 30 years. She stated that she had pain to some degree almost daily. She also indicated that some days she couldn't function because the headache was so bad. After working with this patient, she was completely headache free. That was about 10 or 12 years ago, and she still is headache free.

I have been coming to my office an hour or so early each morning to write this book. Just yesterday, I had a patient come in that had experienced an ATV accident 5 years ago. The imaging was all normal in the ER doctor's eyes, so this patient was released with a prescription for pain pills and muscle relaxers. As time went on, the pain increased. After presenting to the medical doctor again, more medications were prescribed. On one of the subsequent visits back to the medical doctor, more imaging was ordered. Again, no abnormal findings that could explain the pain. Finally, about a year ago, this patient was told that they could inject the area every 2 months for the rest of the patient's life to keep the pain in check.

This patient told me that there would be no healing, and that the accident 5 years ago resulted in life-long pain. However, I did an exam and discovered the cause of the symptoms, and started care. It takes some time to heal, so likely I won't be able to finish this story in this work, but, I repeat, finding the cause of the symptoms and fixing that will allow the body to heal itself.

The human body truly is amazing. Even after all we do to ourselves, we can still heal – it is wonderful!

Contra Indications to Treatment

I don't often get asked about problems that may warrant not treating a patient, but I felt like I would be remiss if I didn't at least try to give the reader a complete explanation. Additionally, there is an alternative that may be considered with certain conditions. I will discuss this alternative at the end of this section.

Probably the number one reason to not perform an inner anal repositioning of the tailbone is because of the presence of anal warts. Anal warts can cause a growth around the anal opening. It is possible, by digitally entering the anal canal with warts present to spread the growth to the inside of the anal canal. Growths inside the anal canal require surgical removal, and it is best to not risk that type of growth. Some of the other conditions are less common, but do occur. The next reasons to not treat are in no particular order, and are not all inclusive.

There may be other reasons to not adjust which I have not listed.

- Old fracture which healed to cause complete fusion of the joints of the tailbone.
- Advanced eating disorders.
- Some cancers.
- Past surgical removal of the tailbone.
- Diseases that cause bleeding disorders.

Obviously, if the joints of the tailbone are completely fused together, the only way to reposition it back is by fracturing the fusion. This re-breaking of the tail bone is not suggested.

Advanced eating disorders cause the entire body to be weakened. Most likely, repositioning the tailbone in these instances, would do little, if any, good because the surrounding tissues would be too weak to hold the tailbone in proper position.

I did have a patient that had recovered from a severe eating disorder, and had married. Her and her husband were trying to conceive with no success. Given her then healthy state, I performed the tailbone adjustment, and her child is now about 15 years old.

Certain cancers often cause the patient to become emancipated much like a person with a severe eating disorder. In the case of cancer, the body is already fighting for its life, and added, less necessary, procedures put added stress on the body's healing processes. This extra stress is not suggested. That said, just like the patient above, when the cancer is gone, and the patient has regained their strength, the adjustment may be very beneficial.

Again, it seems obvious that if there is no tailbone to reposition, then trying to do so would be futile. Therefore, if the patient has undergone surgical tailbone removal (called Coccygectomy) I cannot help them.

When it comes to bleeding disorders, I am not talking about excessive or irregular menstrual bleeding. Bleeding disorders in this instance refers to people that have diseases which cause them to bleed easily and excessively. These diseases range from week blood vessels to a decrease in the needed clotting factors to stop bleeding. There too many possibilities to cover at this point. Although somewhat rare, these diseases do exist, and it is not worth the risk to life of possibly causing a severe anal bleed.

There is one other condition worth mentioning at this point. This condition deals more with the expectations of the patient then the physical condition of the patient. Some ladies just can't get past the thought of having an inner anal procedure performed on them. I fully understand this concern; however, I feel it is, for the most part, un-warranted. At the risk of being somewhat crude and un-caring, let me explain why I feel this concern is un-warranted. First, I use my right index finger when I digitally enter the anal canal. When people defecate, the exiting fecal matter often is greater in diameter then my finger. Because of this, any worries of pain on entrance should be dispelled. Secondly, this is not the only health care treatment involving the anal canal. I remember many years ago my wife had severe nausea after a medical procedure, and the treating physician prescribed a suppository that, once put into the anal canal, was absorbed through the wall lining. (as a side note, this treatment worked very well for her at that time.) Lastly, some women are worried about exposure during the treatment. As I have already mentioned, I do all I can to keep the patient covered in order to keep their integrity intact.

To conclude this section, I will discuss an alternative to digitally entering the anal canal. For some women, this is a viable option although I feel it should only be done when the anal method is not possible. In the case of anal warts, entering the anal canal is not an option, however, the tailbone is located nearly as close to the vaginal opening. It is quite possible to reposition the tailbone by digitally entering the vagina. This technique negates the possibility of spreading the anal warts to the inside of the anal canal. There is a little more tissue between the vaginal wall and the tailbone, so sometimes this method is a little bit uncomfortable. With the amazing results that I have seen with the tailbone adjustment, I feel the vaginal method is a very good option for those that are not candidates for the anal method.

Lastly, some women whom just can't bear the thought of digitally entering the anal canal, opt to have the treatment done using the vaginal canal.

Chapter 7: **What to Expect**

X-Rays Prior to Treatment

When I first opened my practice, and for many years afterwards, I required every patient that was a candidate for a tailbone adjustment to have X-rays. I still believe that the best way to know if someone is truly a candidate, is to obtain X-ray views from the front and from the side of the tailbone. In the last few years, I have performed the tailbone repositioning adjustment on several women without Xrays, and have still gotten the desired results. I came to realize that adjusting the tailbone back to a more normal position works when needed, and does no harm if not needed. Now that doesn't mean I just adjust every woman's tailbone. On the contrary, I make sure that each patient has the symptoms that are consistent with a forward mal-aligned tailbone or I don't adjust. That said, I still prefer to look at a set of X-rays, and I encourage perspective patients to have them taken. The X-rays that are needed are called, weight bearing A to P, and Lateral coccyx views. Don't worry, Your X-ray technician will know how to obtain the proper views. What it means, though, is the patient is standing while the X-rays are taken first from the front and then from the side. I have made it rather simple for a perspective patient to send me their X-rays so that I can review them. After I receive the X-rays, I do my analysis, and return a report to the patient detailing my findings. I also determine if I feel the patient is a candidate for treatment, and include that information with the report. If a patient chooses to not have X-rays, I can make an educated guess after studying their history and symptoms. If you wish to have me look at your case, go to my website and submit the required information.

Sometimes A Little Discomfort

I cannot count the number of tailbone (or coccyx) adjusting procedures I have performed over the years. And, invariably, the lady will say something along the lines of, "oh, is that it?" The adjustment itself is a fairly quick procedure, and is generally pain free for the patient. Occasionally, I have a patient that has experienced an injury severe enough that the forward man-alignment is truly stuck in that position. In those cases, I must apply a little more pressure to get the tailbone to move back. With increased pressure, the chances of increased discomfort or pain go up. Again, I don't often experience this situation, but I never know if it's going to hurt a patient until I actually perform the procedure. Even with those that experience some pain, most say it hurt a little but was no big deal. In the nearly 20 years that I've been doing these adjustments, I have never had a patient experience anything more than the pain described.

I always suggest that the patient have their tailbone adjusted twice. The second adjustment should occur the week following the first adjustment. This ensures that the tailbone stays mobile and functioning in its proper position. Since I have been in practice, I have only had 2 women, that I can remember, that chose to not have the second adjustment because of the pain with the first adjustment. Quite honestly, I feel that even for them the second adjustment would have been beneficial. You see, they had already been through the painful part. With the second adjustment, the tailbone has already been moved so moving it takes much less pressure, and, thus, less discomfort. I can attest to this fact as other ladies have verified that the second adjustment was much better than the first.

Interestingly, one of the 2 patients talked about above was treated recently. This particular patient was experiencing multiple symptoms. The main reason she presented to me was because of vaginal and tailbone pain. This pain was accompanied with severe headaches. She was also experiencing irregular menstrual cycle timing. For example, she would start and finish in 3 days just to start again in 2 weeks and bleed for 10 days. When I performed the tailbone repositioning adjustment, she stated it was painful. I explained to her that the second treatment would likely be less painful, but she chose to not repeat the procedure. I continued to work with the rest of this patient's spine, and, even with only the first tailbone adjustment, she is doing amazingly better. No more headaches, and greatly reduced vaginal and tailbone pain. We don't yet know if she has totally regulated her cycles as enough time has not passed.

Hormonal Response

If I were forced to choose one, and only one, main effect of having a tailbone adjustment, I would have to choose hormonal response. A woman's monthly menstrual cycle is controlled by the cyclic production of her hormones. When I relieve the pressure on the anchoring ligament, by adjusting the tailbone, it also relieves the pressure on the nerves going to the reproductive organs. These organs play a major role in hormone production. While these organs are normalizing, the hormone levels are constantly trying to normalize as well. In the process, the pati9ent experiences highs and lows of the various hormones. These highs and lows affect all women differently, but there are some commonalities among the responses.

One such commonality, as the woman's hormones regulate to more normal levels, is the feelings of emotional ups and downs. She may be happy one minute, and crying for no apparent reason the next minute. She may feel exhilarated then suddenly mad a few moments later. Things that have never bothered her in the past may suddenly be totally annoying to her. With hormonal changes, any, or all, of these symptoms, and others, may occur.

Fortunately, these symptoms usually only last for a couple of weeks to a month. I have had a few patients where it lasted a couple of months, but that is rare. More commonly, women say the hormonal affects were barely noticed. Then, of course, there are the few that don't experience any of the hormonal affects mentioned. All-in-all, I would have to say that most ladies gladly trade a month, or so, of generally mild hormonal symptoms, for the, sometimes, debilitating symptoms they were experiencing prior to treatment. This is especially true with the possibility of no abnormal symptoms afterwards.

Relief

To conclude this short chapter, I will tell you, the reader, the best thing to expect after treatment is relief. The majority of ladies, by and far, just plain feel better. They experience pain relief. They have regular menstrual cycles. They have less headaches. They sleep better. They have more energy. I could name a few more, but I think you get the idea.

It seems in our society that the positive outcomes of various treatments often get lost in the negative "what ifs." Health care providers must cover themselves legally even though those negative results are the few rather than the many. When I write about things that could go wrong, it is for legal reasons. I must do my best to cover every possibility. The reality is most ladies do great. Yes, I do occasionally have some of the negative results arise, but most often the women I work with experience amazing relief from their menstrual related symptoms. In fact, I have so few ladies that don't improve that I have a hard time recalling a story to tell you about. Therefore, no story of a negative.

How about you? If you've read to this point it must be because you have one or more of the conditions I've alluded to. Would you like to correct the problem? Have you tried other treatments with minimal or no results? I've worked with enough patients over the years that I know their trust in healthcare providers can be weakened. I don't blame you if you are still asking yourself, "will this really work for me?" The only way to answer that question is to come to my office and allow me to treat you. I, like other healthcare professionals, can't guarantee results, but I can tell you I have a very high success ratio. The fact is, when a patient doesn't respond to my treatment, I am genuinely surprised. I just get so use to positive results that I have to take a step back, and change my thought process for a bit, when someone doesn't progress as expected.

 In the next chapter, I will tell the true stories of some of the patients I have helped. If you have conditions similar to the ladies in the examples, then it is quite possible you, too, will respond as they did.

Chapter 8: **A Few Success Stories**

Treatment Has A Long History of Success

I know, I know! I promised to tell you some success stories. I will do exactly that, but I felt I should tell you about some of the successes of the doctors before me.

To be quite honest, I really don't know who discovered that the tailbone adjustment had such a positive result. I don't know who the first patient was, or who the doctor was that treated her. What I do know is a couple of un-documented stories told by some of the old doctors that were teaching at the school I attended. One story, in particular, dates back to the 1940's.

While I was at school, one of the teachers was at the end of his teaching career. He was in his 70's, and had been a practicing chiropractor before starting with the school. Interestingly, he was the son of a chiropractor also, and one day he related the following story about his father.

It seems that his father was in his office when his cousin walked through the door. This cousin's wife was experiencing excessive menstrual bleeding each and every cycle. Additionally, they were trying to conceive with no success. The doctor was quite surprised to see this cousin in his office, as this man had openly belittled him and the chiropractic profession in the past. Apparently, however, the couple had exhausted all the other options available at the time. This good doctor explained the tailbone repositioning procedure, and the cousin and his wife went ahead with the treatment. The teacher said that the wife responded just as expected, and that, at the telling of this story, their child was now a grandmother.

I have one other story that is kind of funny. I am certain that for the couple involved it wasn't so funny at the time, but looking back it is worth a giggle. The doctor telling this story had been working with a woman who was experiencing complete irregularity in her menstrual cycles. This woman's husband had been told that his sperm count was not high enough for him to ever father a child. They were just trying to help the wife achieve menstrual health as they were waiting to adopt a child. After revealing this to the doctor, the doctor suggested that perhaps the husband could benefit from the same procedure. The husband was convinced that he was unable to father a child, but agreed to the treatment at his wife's bidding. Well, as the story goes, the wife responded to the treatment as expected, and, as they were waiting for a child to adopt, she became pregnant. The husband was very upset as he was certain there was no way the child was his. His good wife insisted that she had been faithful and that, indeed, he was the father. Sure enough, after the nine-month waiting period, blood tests proved he had fathered his first child.

The main reason I told the above stories is to let the reader know this isn't a new treatment. It is, however, a little used treatment because of the reasons given in an earlier chapter. While at school, I was not the only one who was taught this procedure. The entire class was also taught. But, as I explained earlier, few doctors choose to perform the treatment. Doctors are under constant pressure to not do anything that may cause a law suit, therefore, because the general public is unaware of the tailbone adjustment, they don't want to put themselves at risk. I have never felt that caring for patients the way they needed cared for should be pushed aside due to fear of legal rebuttal. I also believe that patients are smart enough to decide which care they do and do not want to have. Therefore, all I have ever done is explained the treatment to the patient and let them decide. Just as I have done in this book. You, as the reader, should have a good understanding of the treatment at this point. Additionally, you, as the reader, can decide if you want to proceed or not. Because of this approach, I have never in nearly 20 years of practice been sued. I have, however, helped many, many women with their menstrual disorders.

In each of the following sections you will find a true story of a patient that I personally have helped. It is my goal that you will find the stories inspiring, and that perhaps they will restore some hope within you. Just as I helped these ladies, there is a good chance I can help you.

On Her Menstrual Cycle 6 Months
I tell this story first because it is the first tailbone adjustment I performed on a patient. I guess it is human nature to remember the first time you do something. Anyway, I had only been in practice about

3 months when a woman in her late 20's presented to my office.

Her main complaint was low back pain. As I read through her history form, I noticed that she had marked the box indicating irregular menstrual cycles. I asked her to explain why she had marked that box. She commenced to tell me a nearly unbelievable story.

She started by telling me that she had been experiencing heavy menstrual flow for the last 6months. Yes, you read that right – 6 months!! She said that the flow was so heavy that it was, "like diaper rash down there." I asked her what she had done about it up until that point. She proceeded to tell me that her Ob-Gyn thought her hormones were out of balance, so he had prescribed a birth control medication that she was to take for the first 10 days of each month.

I was seeing her about the 15th of the month, and she had just finished her second month of medication a few days earlier. When I asked her if the medications were helping, she stated that on day two of the 10-day prescription the flow nearly stopped. She further explained that by day 10, her bleeding was gone. However, she shrugged her shoulders and said, "on day 11 the bleeding returned with a vengeance."

I need to break away from the story at this point, and tell you what was going through my mind. First, I was experiencing a form of Deja-vu. You see, when I was in college, the professor who taught us how to do the tailbone (or coccyx) adjustment had told very similar stories about some of her patients. I seriously almost looked around to see if I was still in class. Secondly, I had fully decided, like most of the students, that there was no way I was going to stick my finger up anybody's A**! Finally, I had justified this decision by saying that is all well and good for this professor. She was well known for helping women from across the world. She practiced in Davenport, Iowa, but had patients from many countries and most of the United States. I was going to a small town in Utah, and there wouldn't be any need for that type of adjustment. Boy, was I wrong!

Back to my story. My heart went out to this poor woman, so I explained to her about the treatment. Next, I asked if she had injured her tailbone region in the past. Again, her story was eerily similar to the stories the old professor had told. This patient told me she had been living in a bigger city in the mid-west. One weekend, she was attending a backyard barbeque when a van suddenly crashed through the wooded fence that blocked the alley way from the yard. Luckily, she wasn't directly in the path of the van, but the fence did knock her down, and the vehicle ran over her legs. As a result, both of her ankles were broken. Additionally, when she fell, she landed directly on the edge of a concrete flower box with her tailbone.

As you can imagine, the EMT's did a great job getting her to the ER where she was cleared for any life threating injuries. They casted both her ankles; put her in a wheelchair; and sent her home. Over the next few weeks as her ankles healed, she developed a large boil right on top of her tailbone. She recalled the boil being very sore and extremely painful to touch. She said it was difficult for her to sit down due to the pain in caused.

As it turns out, the barbeque she was attending was an engagement party for one of her dearest friends. By the time this patient's ankles were healed, it was time for the wedding. My patient was a bridesmaid for her friend. At the church, there were two wooden staircases that descended on either side of the alter. The bride and her bridesmaids were to walk down one side, and the groom and his groomsmen were to walk down the other side. During the ceremony, while coming down the stairs, this poor woman slipped with her high heels and fell directly on her tailbone bursting that very large, painful boil. I can't even imagine going through that situation. She explained that the blood and pus from the boil soaked her dress and ruined it. She said that the pain and the awful smell forced her to leave the wedding. She continued to explain that the wedding was just a few days prior to her moving to Utah, and that she had started her menstrual cycle during the move and it hadn't stopped since.

I was somewhat torn at this point. Remember my decision? Trust me, I wasn't looking forward to – well you know! But how could I not? My heart went out to this poor woman, and I couldn't do nothing. As it turns out, her husband was with her so we decided to proceed. I obtained the necessary Xrays, and, sure enough, her tailbone (coccyx) was displaced forward. After the described injuries, I was not surprised. I instructed her to undress from the waist down, and to put a gown on. Luckily, at school, the old professor had some dummies that were fairly realistic, so I wasn't totally without experience.

After the initial tailbone adjustment, I gave her time to dress then adjusted the rest of her spine. That was on a Wednesday. I had her return to my office on Friday of the same week. Upon inquiry, she told me that the bleeding had greatly reduced. I again adjusted her spine, and told her to return on Monday of the next week. During Monday's visit, she stated that the bleeding had completely stopped the day before which was Sunday. I continued to care for this patient's spine for about 2 years at which time she moved back to the mid-west. During the 2 years, her menstrual cycle was every 28 days like clockwork. She would come to Utah occasionally during the next few years, and she would always stop to see me, and get adjusted. I would always ask, and she would always confirm, that her menstrual cycle was doing great.

Something that I didn't mention in the above story was the fact that this woman and her husband had one child at that time. They were in hopes of having more children, but the Ob-Gyn had told them if the bleeding didn't stop he would have to do a hysterectomy. You see, the bleeding was threatening this woman's life. She was anemic due to the blood loss, and her body was losing the battle. This couple was understandably saddened by the prospect of having a hysterectomy as that meant no more children.

As a serendipitous close to this story, when I last spoke with this couple, they were the proud parents of 3 beautiful children. I have long forgotten the uncomfortable thought of that first digital anal penetration, but I will never forget the amazing long term positive outcome it had on this good woman's life.

Newlywed Wanting to Get Pregnant
I include this story her because it emphasizes a point that I feel is common in our society. Often, when I work with a woman she has a history of a traumatic, or stressful, event which triggered the irregular menstrual cycle. Or, as in this case, the cessation of a menstrual cycle all together. In this story, the stressful event wasn't a negative, but somewhat of a positive event. Allow me to elaborate.

A friend of mine had recently married a young lady that had been a highly competitive athlete. She played many sports including soccer, basketball, and softball. However, she excelled at long distance running. In fact, she had won many of the running events she entered, and some of the major colleges were trying to recruit her. But, alas, she fell in love, and married my friend instead.

They had been married nearly a year when she visited my office. She had heard that I may be able to help her with irregular menstrual cycles. During my initial consultation, I discovered that this young woman had not had a menstrual cycle in about 8 months, and that the one she did have was the only one in the last couple of years.

You see, when a female athlete competes at a high level, it is common for them to not have a menstrual cycle. Their bodies adapt to the greater physical demands and conserve energy in any way it can. This commonly includes putting menstrual cycles on hold. I have seen this in several female patients. In this case, though, her cycles didn't return after she quit competing.

Now, I have had some ladies tell me how wonderful it would be to not have to deal with a menstrual cycle every month, but this young couple wanted to have a child. If a woman doesn't have normal menstrual cycles, it is very difficult for her to conceive.

I asked al the inquiring questions about past traumatic events to no avail. This patient could not recall any injuries. Her stress was the highly competitive training and running she had done. I believe there are many ladies in this world that have experienced similar symptoms.

I explained the internal coccyx (tailbone) adjustment to her and her husband, and they decided to move forward with the treatment. Interestingly, her body was so used to not having a normal cycle, that it took about 3 months before her body was functioning as expected.

Of course, I wouldn't be telling this story if there wasn't a happy ending. As you should have guessed, their baby is now about 10 years old and has two younger siblings. Again, part of my goal in telling this story is to point out that sometimes seemingly normal events can stress our systems. With a little help administered the correct way, our bodies can heal and move to a healthier state.

Sitting On Bleachers

I live in a small town in rural Utah where farming and ranching are a way of life. Indeed, many of my past patients are fully dependent on farming and ranching as their sole source of income. As is common in most such communities, rodeo goes along naturally with the lifestyle. This next story is about one such woman and her experience with the rodeo.

This lady did not actually compete in the rodeo, but she had family that did. More specifically, her cousin was a team roper competing at the high school and college levels. This patient and her cousin had grown up together and were very supportive of each other. Although she had married, and at the time had two small children, she still liked to go to her cousin's rodeo events. The seating area for friends and families to watch the rodeo events was composed of bleachers much like those found in many high school gymnasiums.

When this patient first presented to me, her and her husband were trying to have a third child. She explained that her menstrual cycles had become irregular and very painful. She also complained of migraine headaches just prior to and during her cycle. Although I asked all the questions I could think of, we could not discover, at that time, why her cycles had so dramatically changed for the worst. None the-less, I explained the treatment, and obtained X-rays. Sure enough, her tailbone was displaced forward. Again, we could find no explanation as to how this had happened. She followed through with the treatment, and in a short time became pregnant. However, this is not the end of the story.

Her pregnancy and delivery went as expected, and her third child was a beautiful, bouncing baby girl. After recovering from delivery, and adapting to life with her now 3 children, she went back to some of the activities she enjoyed. One such activity was going to her cousin's rodeo events.

A little over a year after her third child was born, she came back to my office with the same symptoms as before. However, this time she knew what had happened. She went on to explain that one day, while she was sitting on the bleachers, she felt the pressure push her coccyx forward. She asked if I would repeat

the procedure which I did. Sure enough, just as
before, her symptoms abated, and her menstrual
cycles returned to normal. She also quit having the
migraine headaches. As a side note, to finish this
story, she is now the mother of 4, and carries a
cushioned bleachers chair with her to the rodeos.

Cramps Stop

If I were to guess, I would say that severe menstrual
cramping is probably the most common menstrual
irregularity. I know that many women have cramps
during their menstrual cycle, but severe cramps are
not normal. I also believe that, given the choice,
women with severe cramps would like to have them
gone. This next story tells of such a case.

This patient was actually an 18-year-old girl. For
some reason, she had experienced severe menstrual
cramping since shortly after beginning her menstrual
cycles. By the time she presented to me, she was
having cramping so severe that when they started she
stayed home. The pain made It so she couldn't
function. The only relief she could find was to lay
down with a heating pad placed over her abdomen
and pelvic regions.

I had treated this patient's mother for an unrelated condition, and her mother hoped I would be able to help her. After explaining to her the treatment to move her coccyx back to a more normal position, she said she was willing to do anything to get rid of the severe cramps. I obtained X-rays, and scheduled her for treatment.

On the appointed day, and at the appointed hour, she didn't show up. Understanding the potentially compromising nature of the treatment, I assumed this young girl had changed her mind. A little later that day, her mother called to see if I could still see her that day. As it turned out, we had an opening in a few minutes, so she and her mother came in. They went on to explain that the patient had started her menstrual cycle that morning, and she just didn't feel like doing anything but lay in bed.
I explained that her being on her menstrual cycle shouldn't affect the administration of my treatment. Further, I suggested that, because she was already in my office, we should go ahead and treat her right then. She apprehensively agreed, so I had her dress in a gown.

Now, after I adjust a patient's coccyx (tailbone), I always leave the room to allow the patient to re-dress. Additionally, after washing my hands, I return to the room to adjust the remainder of the patient's spine. As you can imagine, re-dressing and washing hands only takes a few minutes. Well, that few minutes was all it took. In that short span of time, when I returned to the room, her cramps were gone! She stated that she was still a little sore, but the severe cramps had completely stopped. I was as surprised as she was. With all the ladies I've treated over the years, she experienced the fastest results.

That family moved from the area shortly afterwards, and I was unable to monitor this patient's progress of the next few years. Then one day this young mother walked through my office door to tell me thanks. At that time, the only other time I've seen her, she was still doing fine.

I don't expect patients to respond that quickly, but some patients do have what is considered an unexplainably rapid recovery. As I mentioned earlier in this book, it usually takes a little time for the healing process to complete.

Conclusion

20 Years

As a close to this chapter, and ultimately the ending of the book, I have a question for you. Have you ever visited a medical specialist? If so, why? I guess I should phrase my question more to why did you go, and why did you go to that specialist? I'm certain that the answer is because, being a specialist, this person is focused on helping with just the condition you had. Additionally, they are a specialist because of the experience they have. Let's be honest, whatever the condition you were experiencing was, that prompted a visit to a specialist, your general medical practitioner could likely treat. Most general practitioners are versed in all the various ailments that people suffer from.

The reason I'm pointing out the above is because going to a specialist is the best way to get specialized care. The general practitioner likely will not find the detailed problems specific to you. Could he or she treat you? Yes, but would it be the best treatment?

When it comes to treating patients with a forward misplaced coccyx, most chiropractors are familiar with the treatment. And, honestly, they could treat you. However, I've been doing these treatments for nearly 20 years on many, many women. I have had amazing results.

If you would like to have me treat you, or have me look at your case, go to my website www.Naturalflowforwomen.com to find out how I can do that for you.

I would like to thank you for your time in reading this book, and may all your future menstrual cycles be normal and healthy.

J. Dean Fitzgerald, DC

Natural Flow:

- Free One-On-One Consultation
  Spend 20-30 minutes to discuss how we can help you
- Everyone who applies for a consultation receives a gift

4 WAYS TO REGISTER

Mobile Text
Text to: 58885 your name and email with the keyword "**Flow**"

Voice
Call 866-603-3995 PIN # 149400

Web
www.bonus.Naturalflowforwomen.com

QR Code